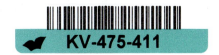

Case Presentations in
Accident and Emergency Medicine

Titles in the series

Case Presentations in Accident and Emergency Medicine

Case Presentations in Arterial Disease

Case Presentations in Clinical Geriatric Medicine

Case Presentations in Endocrinology and Diabetes

Case Presentations in Gastrointestinal Disease

Case Presentations in General Surgery

Case Presentations in Heart Disease (Second Edition)

Case Presentations in Medical Ophthalmology

Case Presentations in Neurology

Case Presentations in Obstetrics and Gynaecology

Case Presentations in Otolaryngology

Case Presentations in Paediatrics

Case Presentations in Renal Medicine

Case Presentations in Respiratory Medicine

Titles in preparation

Case Presentations in Anaesthesia and Intensive Care

Case Presentations in Psychiatry

Case Presentations in Urology

Case Presentations in Accident and Emergency Medicine

Francis Morris, MB, BS, MRCP, FRCS(A&E)
Consultant in Accident and Emergency Medicine,
Northern General Hospital, Sheffield

Fionna Moore, BSc, MB, BS, FRCS, FRCS(Ed)
Consultant in Accident and Emergency Medicine,
University College Hospital, London

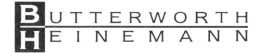

Butterworth-Heinemann Ltd
Linacre House, Jordan Hill, Oxford OX2 8DP

$\mathcal{R}$ A member of the Reed Elsevier group

OXFORD   LONDON   BOSTON
MUNICH   NEW DELHI   SINGAPORE   SYDNEY
TOKYO   TORONTO   WELLINGTON

First published 1993
Reprinted 1994

British Library Cataloguing in Publication Data
Morris, Francis
   Case Presentations in Accident and Emergency
   Medicine – (Case Presentation Series)
   I. Title   II. Moore, Fionna   III. Series
   616.02

   ISBN 0 7506 1378 5

Library of Congress Cataloging in Publication Data
Morris, Francis.
   Case Presentations in accident and emergency medicine/Francis
   Morris, Fionna Moore.
   p.   cm.
   Includes bibliographical references and index.
   ISBN 0 7506 1378 5
   1. Emergency medicine – Case studies.   I. Moore, Fionna.
   II. Title.
   [DNLM: 1. Accidents – case studies.   2. Emergencies – case studies.
   3. Emergency Medicine – case studies.   WB 105 M875c]
   RC86.7.M65
   616.02′5–dc20   92–49711
                                          CIP

Composition by Genesis Typesetting, Laser Quay, Rochester, Kent
Printed and bound in Great Britain by
Biddles Ltd, Guildford and King's Lynn

Preface

This book contains sixty or so case histories all based upon real patients that we have seen. The format for each case history has been standardized.

For each, the relevant history and examination findings are given and you are asked to answer a number of questions on this information.

Many of the common medical emergencies are covered, as are some of the medical problems which are peculiar to accident and emergency work.

We have attempted to provide a balanced cross-section of accident and emergency work in the case histories although limitations of space have prevented it from being comprehensive.

We hope that you will find the case history style of this book both an informative and enjoyable introduction to emergency medicine.

FPM & FPM

Acknowledgement

We would like to extend our thanks to Ellie Carr and William Foulkes without whom this book would not be written.

To our colleagues Peter Driscoll, Andrew Cope, Stephen Hawes, David Skinner, Arvinder Sadana and Edwin Rajarajan, all in the field of accident and emergency medicine who gave willingly of their time and criticism.

We would also like to thank the following doctors who were able to give specialist advice for particular case histories: Kevin Jones (General Medicine and Respiratory Medicine), Philip Robinson (ENT), Robert Greenbaum (Cardiology), Peter Frecker (General Surgery), John Brazier (Ophthalmology) and Katriona Erskine (Gynaecology).

FPM & FPM

Case 1

A 54-year-old woman presented with a headache. At 10:00 that morning she suddenly developed a severe left frontotemporal headache, and promptly vomited three times. She described this episode as the worst headache that she had ever had. There had been no aura or visual disturbance, though she felt quite dizzy. She was currently taking pizotifen as a prophylactic agent as she suffered quite frequent attacks of migraine. She described a typical attack of migraine as the sudden onset of a unilateral headache, nausea and photophobia, but vomiting was unusual. For the past 2 years she had taken atenolol for hypertension. There was no other relevant history.

On examination:

- Irritable
- Alert and orientated, time, place and person
- Pyrexial 37.8°C, pulse 50/min, blood pressure 170/100 mmHg
- Fundi normal, no neck stiffness, no focal neurological signs
- Symmetrically brisk reflexes with down going plantars
- The rest of the examination was normal

Questions

1 What is the differential diagnosis?
2 Describe your management?

Answer

1 Differential diagnosis

Migraine would be an obvious diagnosis given her past medical history, but why, has a woman with long-standing migraine come to hospital with another attack? Obviously there is something different about his headache compared with the others. Is it that it is just more severe? The sudden onset of a headache and vomiting in a hypertensive woman should always suggest the possibility of subarachnoid haemorrhage. This condition is characterized by sudden headache, usually occipital or frontal, associated with vomiting and transient altered level of consciousness. Some patients remain completely alert, while others are rendered immediately unconscious. Neck stiffness, and photophobia are variable symptoms. Most commonly the underlying pathology is a ruptured cerebral aneurysm. Other less common causes of subarachnoid haemorrhage are bleeding from an arteriovenous malformation, extension of an intracerebral bleed to involve the subarachnoid space, anticoagulants and blood dyscrasias.

Helpful confirmatory signs which must be looked for include:

- Meningeal irritation (neck stiffness may take up to 24 h before it becomes obvious)
- Altered level of consciousness
- Photophobia
- Mild pyrexia – due to the inflammatory response to blood in the subarachnoid space
- Retinal or subhyaloid haemorrhages

Subarachnoid haemorrhage is associated with the release of sympathetic amines which may give rise to changes in the electrocardiogram (ST depression), myocardial ischaemia and occasionally infarction. Neurogenic pulmonary oedema may also occur.

Meningitis should always be considered in the differential diagnosis and a lumbar puncture is mandatory when there is doubt. The onset of the headache in meningitis is typically gradual over several hours rather than explosive in nature, though atypical presentations are well recognized.

2 Management

This woman should be nursed lying flat, and referred to the duty medical team for exclusion of a subarachnoid haemorrhage.

When there is an altered level of consciousness the airway should be maintained at all times and 60% oxygen supplied via a Venturi mask.

An anaesthetist, and the medical registrar should be called immediately for a patient in a coma (Glasgow coma scale < 8) or with a respiratory rate of less than 10/min. These patients may need assisted ventilation. This will ensure adequate oxygenation and allow controlled hyperventilation to lower the P_{CO_2} and thereby help in combating rising intracranial pressure.

The investigation of choice is computed tomographic (CT) scanning. The majority of patients with subarachnoid haemorrhage will have a positive CT scan (blood demonstrated in the subarachnoid space). The localization of this blood may give an indication of the site of the bleed.

Early neurosurgical consultation is necessary. Lumbar puncture is necessary if the CT scan is negative or if meningitis cannot be excluded. This procedure should be performed by an experienced doctor and it is vital that the CSF is examined for xanthachromia – this may not be present until 6 h after the bleed.

If a subarachnoid haemorrhage is confirmed then the patient may benefit from nimodipine (calcium antagonist) which has been shown to reduce the incidence of delayed ischaemic deficits (60 mg/4 h is the recommended dose).

Outcome

A CT scan confirmed the presence of blood in the subarachnoid space. The patient remained alert, however, neck stiffness was noted 12 h after admission. She was referred to the neurosurgical team who undertook arteriography and elective surgery to clip the aneurysm of the left middle cerebral artery at 10 days.

Further notes on subarachnoid haemorrhage

Rupture of a vascular aneurysm is the most common established cause of spontaneous subarachnoid haemorrhage. Although these aneurysms are found in all age groups, with a women to men ratio of 3:2, the peak incidence of rupture is 40–60 years of age. There is an association between aneurysm and coarctation of the aorta, polycystic kidney disease and connective tissue disorders.

The causes of non-aneurysmal subarachnoid haemorrhage have been listed above, but in up to 20% of cases no cause can be determined.

Fontanarosa (1989), reviewed the presenting features of 109 spontaneous subarachnoid haemorrhages presenting to an Accident and Emergency department. His findings contained the following salient observations:

1 Over 50% were involved in some sedentary activity such as sleeping when they first noticed the symptoms, and less than 25% were known to be involved in exertional activities.
2 The commonest presenting symptoms were headache and vomiting with a significant minority giving a history of brief loss of consciousness. Sudden onset of confusion, or coma were found in 28% and 36% respectively, but in 36% the patient was alert.
3 The clinical findings at presentation revealed that only 35% had obvious neck stiffness, this is an important fact to remember; 32% were noted to be hypertensive, and only 5% had retinal haemorrhages.
4 Of the 109 patients the Accident and Emergency staff made a correct diagnosis in 93 cases, and in the remaining 16 the commonest erroneous diagnoses were cerebral infarction, hypertensive crisis, or a generalized viral illness.

While the majority of patients do not have focal signs, they can occur. Pressure from an expanding clot, or haemorrhage into the brain substance, together with pressure on cranial nerves can give rise to focal symptoms and signs. This may give the examiner some clue as to the probable sites of the aneurysm. The incidence at various sites is approximately:

Internal carotid circulation	40%
Anterior carotid circulation	35%
Middle cerebral circulation	20%
Posterior circulation	5%

Rupture at the various sites give rise to the following signs:

Anterior cerebral circulation:

- Asymptomatic before rupture.
- Typical features of subarachnoid haemorrhage and an associated confusional state.

Middle cerebral circulation:

- Asymptomatic before rupture.
- Typical features of subarachnoid haemorrhage and associated hemiparesis, hemisensory loss, dysphasia and seizures.

Posterior cerebral circulation:

- Headache and progressive III nerve signs before rupture and typical symptoms after rupture.

The main differential diagnosis when there are focal signs, include cerebral infarction/haemorrhage, but focal migraine is a diagnosis of exclusion. Several studies have pointed to the fact that up to 60% of patients presenting with subarachnoid haemorrhage have had a 'warning leak' in the previous days, weeks or months. Therefore, the onset of sudden headache in a patient not known to suffer recurrent headaches, especially if associated with vomiting should be treated with suspicion.

Practice points

1 Any patient presenting with sudden headache with or without vomiting may have had a subarachnoid haemorrhage.
2 Neck stiffness may be absent at presentation.
3 Subarachnoid haemorrhage should be included in the differential diagnosis of any patient who presents in coma.

References

Kennedy, H. J. (1985) *Emergencies in Medicine.* Blackwell, Oxford
Fontanarosa, P. B. (1989) Recognition of SAH. *Annals of Emergency Medicine,* **1,** 1199

Case 2

A man aged 19 years was working on a building site when he thought he got something in his right eye, he rubbed it, and then rinsed it out with water. Rather than improving the situation, this made it worse. His eye watered profusely, he had an intense foreign body sensation, and was photophobic. He presented to the Accident and Emergency department. He had no history of previous eye problems, or other serious medical problems.

On examination:

- Right eye red and injected
- Visual acuity: right 6/12; left 6/18 uncorrected. (He had not brought his glasses with him)

Questions

1 What further history is necessary?
2 How do you interpret the visual acuity results?
3 What would your management be if you found a metallic corneal foreign body?
4 What would your management be if you failed to find a foreign body?

Answers

1 What further history is necessary?

When there is a history of a potential foreign body in the eye it is extremely important to ask about the exact circumstances of the incident. A history which involves hammering, metal on metal, or metal on stone, drilling, working on a lathe or grinding may indicate the possibility of a penetrating eye injury. High velocity particles of metal, and occasionally stone or glass can penetrate the eye leaving an entry wound which can appear trivial and the possibility of penetration overlooked if the history is not appreciated.

Similarly patients involved in road traffic accidents where the windscreen shatters are at high risk from penetrating eye injuries from glass.

2 Visual acuity

It is vitally important to measure the visual acuity in both eyes in all patients with eye injuries. Visual acuity is recorded using a Snellen's test card. The smallest type line on which most of the letters are read correctly is recorded. Visual acuity is expressed as a fraction which can range from 6/60 (the top letter on the chart) to 6/6 or better. 6/6 is considered normal.

The use of a pinhole corrects for refractive errors. Thus, if a patient's diminished visual acuity does not improve with a pinhole, an organic disease should be suspected. Although the reduction in visual acuity may be long standing, it should always be assumed to be acute when a patient presents with an injury, or new condition. When a patient's vision is so poor that they are unable to read any of the type print on a Snellen chart, then acuity should be documented in terms of counting fingers (CF), hand movements (HM) or to perceive light (PL).

Note: If the patient presents with a painful eye and finds it too difficult to keep open to mesure the visual acuity then instill local anaesthetic drops to ensure you get a measurement.

3 What is your management if you find a metallic corneal foreign body?

Corneal foreign bodies are usually easily seen with the naked eye. Commonly they are found on the lower half of the cornea because of the reflex turning up of the eye with closure of the eyelids on the awareness of an approaching object.

With magnification (ideally a slit lamp) the eye should be examined for other potential foreign bodies, or evidence of a scleral or corneal wound which might indicate a penetrating injury. The upper eyelid should always be inverted to exclude an additional subtarsal foreign body.

Having excluded other pathology the corneal foreign body should be removed. The cornea should be anaesthetized with local anaesthetic and the foreign body removed with a 25 gauge needle. This procedure is not without its hazards. Before starting, the situation should be explained to the patient to ensure full cooperation. It is important that the patient's head remains in a fixed position, and that they fix on a distant object to prevent eye movements. The needle should be attached to a 1 ml or 2 ml syringe as this makes it more manoeuvrable. The hand holding the syringe should rest on the patient's cheek, or nose, (depending on the eye) so that the hand and therefore the needle moves with the patient's head if there is a sudden jolt. The needle should be advanced at an oblique angle and the foreign body dislodged from the cornea, and then removed with a cotton wool bud. Invariably a metallic foreign body leaves behind a rust ring, which should ideally be removed at the same time again by gently loosening it with the needle. If this is too extensive, or extends too deep for confident removal, the patient should be referred to the ophthalmology team.

Any patient unable to tolerate the thought of the procedure and who does not keep still, or patients with deeply bedded foreign bodies should likewise be referred.

Once removed the patient should be given antibiotic drops for 5 days. The patient should be advised that the defect in the cornea left by the foreign body will likely give rise to mild symptoms over the next 24 h.

Patients from an environment where a high velocity particle cannot be excluded should have an orbital radiograph. A single screening AP film of both orbits should be taken initially. Any suspicious abnormality can be localized with additional films. Two further AP films with the eye looking up and then down demonstrates whether any potential foreign body moves with the eye. A lateral film can further aid to localize the foreign body. Remember that metal corneal foreign bodies should be removed before the radiographs are taken, as they can cause confusion. A negative radiograph does not exclude a penetrating eye injury, or a retained foreign body, particularly when glass is involved.

4 What is your management if no foreign body is found?

When no foreign body is found, never forget to evert the upper lid to exclude a subtarsal foreign body (this is ophthalmologist's equivalent of a rectal examination).

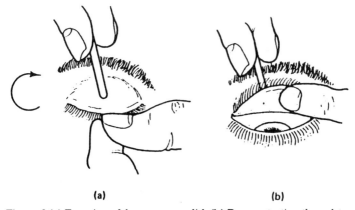

(a)   **(b)**

Figure 1 (a) Eversion of the upper eyelid. (b) Demonstrating the subtarsal conjunctiva (From Brown, A. F. T. (1992) *Accident and Emergency: Diagnosis and Management*. 2nd edn. Butterworth-Heinemann, Oxford)

It is possible that the intense watering and blinking associated with a foreign body has helped to dislodge it, and a small corneal abrasion is the only evidence left of its presence. When examination of the eye to white light reveals no evidence of a foreign body a thorough search for a corneal or scleral laceration should be made. The addition of fluorescein is then necessary, and the eye should be examined under blue light. Fluorescein stains epithelial defects bright green when viewed under blue light and therefore highlights small abrasions caused by a foreign body or eye rubbing, or corneal lacerations. The appearance of multiple vertical linear epithelial damage (scratches) on the cornea are indicative of a subtarsal foreign body. This may have been washed out, if no subtarsal foreign body is evident.

Corneal abrasions are treated with chloramphenicol drops, and eye padding. All but the very large ones will heal within 48 h. Again patients engaged in a high risk occupation for high velocity foreign bodies should have an orbital radiograph.

Any patient with a corneal or scleral laceration, or with a suspected foreign body on the radiograph should be sent directly to the ophthalmologist, as it will be necessary to examine the posterior segment as well as the anterior segment. All patients with corneal foreign bodies, or abrasion sustained at work should be advised about the need to use protective glasses while engaged in high risk occupations.

Outcome

In this patient, the history was not suggestive of a high velocity penetrating injury. Visual acuity was 6/6 in both eyes when corrected with a pinhole. The foreign body was removed along with the rust ring. He was given an eye pad and chloramphenicol eye drops. On review after 48 h he was asymptomatic and the corneal lesion had healed.

Practice points

1 Always assess visual acuity, and if necessary use a pinhole to correct for refractive errors. Use local anaesthetic drops if discomfort interferes with accurate measurement.
2 Always take a full history, bearing in mind the possibility of penetrating injury.
3 Perform an orbital radiograph if the history is suggestive of penetrating injury even in the absence of clinical evidence.

Reference

Bron, A. J. and Davey, C. C. (1987) *The Unquiet Eye*. Glaxo Laboratories Ltd, Greenford
Brown, A. F. T. (1992) *Accident and Emergency: Diagnosis and Management*. 2nd edn. Butterworth-Heinemann, Oxford

Case 3

A 10-year-old girl presented with lower abdominal pain. It had started 9 h previously at 01:00, and had woken her from sleep. The pain was initially intermittent and was felt 'all over' her abdomen. She was unable to sleep because of the pain and was nauseated. She was troubled with urinary frequency, and was constantly going to the toilet, but she only passed small quantities of urine each time and it did not burn or sting. At 06:00 she was aware that the pain was more severe in nature, and was no longer intermittent. She now experienced the pain in the right iliac fossa and suprapubic area. This was worse with movement, and did not radiate anywhere.

Over the next 3 h the pain increased in intensity and she vomited twice. The urinary frequency had not abated. There was no diarrhoea.

She was brought to Accident and Emergency by her parents. They confirmed that she had been well recently and that there had been no significant past medical history and she had not reached menarche.

On examination:

- Flushed, pyrexial 38.2°C
- Dry mouth, throat normal, chest clear
- Coughing exacerbated the pain
- Abdomen – tender, and rebound tenderness in the right iliac fossa and suprapubic area
- Rectal examination: tender on the right, bowel sounds normal
- No renal angle tenderness
- Urine – none available for analysis

Questions

1 What is the diagnosis?
2 What is your management?

Answers

1 The presenting symptoms of lower abdominal pain, urinary frequency, and the finding of fever and suprapubic tenderness in a 10-year-old girl may all suggest that a lower urinary tract infection is the diagnosis. However, the type and severity of the pain might be suggestive of an alternative diagnosis. It is interesting to note that, of patients with urinary trace infections that do present to hospital, only 5% of them do so within 12 h of the onset of their symptoms.

Many of this girl's presenting symptoms and signs are compatible with appendicitis. Indeed the nature of this girl's pain, the initial poorly localized, colicky pain which then moved to become a well localized continuous pain, is highly suggestive of this diagnosis. The change in the site of the pain which is typical of appendicitis is due to the fact that an inflamed appendix initially gives rise to mid-gut colic. This is a diffuse, colicky pain centred around the umbilicus or felt 'all over', which then moves to the site of the appendix when peritoneal inflammation becomes pronounced. I say to the site of the appendix, rather than the right iliac fossa because, although in the majority of cases inflammation localizes there, occasionally it can be felt in the suprapubic area, the left iliac fossa (with a pelvic appendix) or up towards the right hypochondrium with a retrocaecal appendix.

Urinary symptoms may be present if the inflamed appendix irritates the ureter or bladder (occasionally producing both red and white blood cells in the urine) and are found in a significant minority of cases (6%).

The symptoms and signs of fever, facial flushing, nausea and vomiting are not helpful in discriminating between the two conditions. However, the rebound tenderness, and the right-sided tenderness elicited on rectal examination are much more suggestive of appendicitis than a urinary tract infection.

2 The patient should be referred to the duty surgical team for assessment and a possible appendicectomy once a urinary tract infection has been excluded.

Outcome

With intravenous fluid administration a urine sample was obtained which was normal on microscopy.

An inflamed appendix was removed at operation.

Further notes

Points to remember when making the diagnosis of appendicitis:

- Patients often present with right lower quadrant pain. The apparent predilection for abdominal pain to present in this site, is partly due to the fact that both patients and general practitioners are very aware of the possibility of appendicitis and therefore are more likely to refer such patients to hospital.
- Helpful clinical features (after de Dombal (1991) that are suggestive of appendicitis are:

  1 Site of pain:
  Pain which is initially intermittent that moves from the midline to the right lower quadrant. The pain is well localized and constant here.
  2 Aggravating factors:
  Movement and coughing give rise to pain.
  3 Constitutional upset:
  Nausea, vomiting, and anorexia are all usually present.
  4 Patient is flushed, and has a low grade pyrexia.
  5 Focal tenderness is found in the right lower quadrant.
  Patients with diffuse tenderness are less likely to have appendicitis, as are those with focal tenderness remote from the right lower quadrant.
  6 Both rebound and guarding are present.
  7 Rectal examination:
  Localized tenderness on the right side.

If more than two of these features are present the patient should be admitted to hospital for observation. Patients with four features or more warrant appendicectomy.

The white cell count is helpful when raised though a normal result does not exclude the diagnosis.

Practice points

1 Always examine the urine of patients with suspected appendicitis under a microscope.
2 A full gynaecological history and a pelvic examination are necessary in women of child-bearing age who are thought to have appendicitis. Both pelvic inflammatory disease and ectopic pregnancy can cause diagnostic difficulty.
3 Many of the typical features of appendicitis may not be present in the elderly or the very young.

Cautionary tale
An 18-month-old Bengali female child was brought by her parents because she had a fever for 3 days. On the second day of the illness the child had vomited several times, and had episodes of diarrhoea. On examination the child looked flushed but well, and was actually drinking some milk when first seen. The abdomen was completely rigid. At operation a perforated appendix was removed.

Reference

de Dombal, F. T. (1991) *Diagnosis of Acute Abdominal Pain.* 2nd edn. Churchill Livingstone, Edinburgh

Case 4

You are asked to see a woman of 25 years, who came to the Accident and Emergency department with a deterioration in the control of her asthma. She had been given a nebulizer, and now feels much better and as a consequence wants to return home. The following history is obtained.

She had been getting progressively more short of breath over the past 3 days. It had started with a sore throat and a cough. She had been sleeping poorly, and has had chest tightness in the morning. She is a long-standing mild asthmatic, normally controlled upon salbutamol and beclomethasone inhalers. She is a smoker, and is on the oral contraceptive pill. Other than mild eczema and hayfever there is no other significant history.

On examination:

- Well
- Apyrexial
- Able to speak in sentences
- Respiratory rate 20/min, pulse 120/min, blood pressure 110/70 mmHg, no pulsus paradoxus
- Using accessory muscles of respiration
- Some intercostal recession
- Bilateral wheeze
- No clinical pneumothorax
- Heart sounds normal
- Abdomen soft
- No evidence of deep venous thrombosis
- Peak flow 220 l/min (pre-nebulizer 130 l/min)

Questions

1 What are the important factors to elicit in the history of an asthmatic?
2 How do you assess the severity of an asthma attack?
3 What is the management of acute severe asthma?
4 Which patients do you admit?

Answers

1 Essential aspects of the history are:

(a) The length of time the patient has been asthmatic, and the frequency and severity of previous attacks, e.g. the number of acute attacks per year, how quickly these symptoms deteriorate, whether hospital admission was necessary, and particularly whether artificial ventilation has been necessary previously.

(b) Usual maintenance therapy: is this taken regularly, as prescribed, and is it adequate to control the symptoms? Or is the patient always wheezy, has a decreased exercise capacity, or troublesome nocturnal symptoms?

(c) What normally precipitates an attack, e.g. exercise, emotion, infection?
What precipitated this attack?
Was it failure to take normal medication?

2 Patients present to Accident and Emergency when their normal maintenance therapy is inadequate to control their symptoms. Often patients notice that relief from symptoms after using their bronchodilator becomes increasingly short lived. Some patients fail to notice the severity of their symptoms and present in extremis. Both patients and their

relatives tend to underestimate the severity of an attack. Grave signs on presentation, representing life-threatening emergencies are:

- Cyanosis
- Altered consciousness, confusion
- Exhaustion
- A silent chest on examination
- High P_{CO_2} in a breathless patient,
  Low P_{O_2} or pH despite 60% oxygen
- Bradycardia

All the above indicate the need for artificial ventilation. The medical team and the anaesthetist should be called immediately.

For less severely affected patients an assessment of their condition *before* the nebulizer is necessary. The diagnosis of *acute severe asthma* can be inferred from:

(a) The change in the patient's exercise tolerance from normal, and
(b) from the clinical criteria listed below:

a *Exercise tolerance*
  Grade I: Able to carry out normal activities with difficulty

  Grade II: Confined to a chair or bed but able to get up with moderate difficulty (IIa) or with great difficulty (IIb)

  Grade III: Totally confined to a chair or bed

  Grade IV: Moribund

Greater than IIa, suggests acute severe asthma.

b *Signs*
  The presence of the following signs indicate acute severe asthma, and should be sought in all patients:

  - Inability to complete sentences due to breathlessness.
  - Using accessory muscles of respiration, tracheal tug, and intercostal recession.
  - Respiratory rate above 25/min.
  - Pulse rate above 110/min.
  - Palpable pulsus paradox, or an inspiratory fall in systolic blood pressure of greater than 10 mmHg.
  - Peak expiratory flow rate of less than 40% of the predicted value, or best obtainable value if known. (Otherwise less than 200 l/min would be indicative of an acute severe attack in most people.)
  - Arterial blood gases should be taken in any patient with the signs of acute severe attack, as invariably they will be hypoxic due to ventilation/perfusion mismatch. Many patients will have a good response to an initial nebulizer, and will consequently feel much better. It is important to remember that this improvement will be short lived, and post nebulizer assessments can be very misleading. The initial assessment prior to the nebulizer delivers the most useful

information on which to base management decisions. Therefore never be tempted to prescribe a nebulized bronchodilator without assessing the patient first.

3 Initial management should include the following:

a Clinical assessment.
b All patients should be given 60% oxygen via Venturi mask (never 24 or 28%).
c 5 mg of terbutaline/salbutamol via nebulizer in oxygen.
d Estimation of arterial blood gases.
e 30 mg of prednisolone orally (200 mg of hydrocortisone i.v. if unable to tolerate oral administration).
f Chest radiograph necessary to exclude a pneumothorax, or focal consolidation.
g Never sedate, strong verbal reassurance should be used.
h Antibiotics are rarely indicated.

Asthmatics often produce green sputum, due to the high eosinophil production, and this is not an indication for treatment, but a fever and chest radiograph changes are.

Response in terms of peak flow, paradox, pulse and respiratory rate etc. should be documented. Additional therapy may be required if the initial response is inadequate.

Additional therapy

a Patients with the signs and symptoms of acute severe asthma that fail to respond to initial therapy will need further aggressive management.

- Call the medical team.
- Continue to give 60% oxygen at all times. Repeat the nebulizer of β_2-agonist, and add 500 μg of ipratropium bromide to the nebulizer solution.
- Give intravenous aminophylline (5 mg/kg over 30 min), unless the patient has been taking oral theophyllines at home as maintenance therapy. In that case give an intravenous β_2-agonist, e.g. salbutamol 200 μg or terbutaline 250 μg over 10 min.
- If the patient develops any of the imminently life-threatening features, as tabulated above:
  call the anaesthetist.
- Repeat peak flow estimations, and monitor blood pressure, pulse and respiratory rate.
- Repeat blood gases.

Arterial blood gases

The hypoxia associated with acute asthma is corrected to some degree by increasing the inspired O_2 concentration. Normally patients with acute asthma will have a low $P_{a}CO_2$ as a consequence of hyperventilation, and if the $P_{a}CO_2$ is normal or raised this is a grave sign.

Ventilation is necessary when (on 60% oxygen):

$P_{a}O_2 < 8\,kPa$
$P_{a}CO_2 > 6.5\,kPa$
$pH < 7.2$

4 Nearly 2000 asthmatics die each year, and many of these have seen a medical practitioner within the previous 48 h, emphasizing the tendency to underestimate the severity of attacks. It is safer to assume that all asthmatics should be admitted unless a very good case can be made for discharging them.

Guidelines for discharging patients with asthma

- On initial assessment the patient had none of the signs of acute severe asthma, i.e. peak flow > 200 l/min etc.
- Response to treatment has been good, i.e. peak flow > 75% of known, or predicted PFR.
- All patients have a short course of oral prednisolone (30 mg a day for 7 days in the first instance), inhaled steroids and bronchodilator (ensure technique is adequate).
- Patients should see their general practitioners within 36 h, with a letter detailing treatment and peak flow estimations. The general practitioner will reduce the steroids according to the patient's response.
- Hospital follow-up is arranged.
- If in doubt admit the patient.

Remember that asthma deteriorates during the night. Be very circumspect about discharging patients home late evening or early morning.

Outcome

This woman has some features of acute severe asthma and although clinically improving, her peak flow after the first nebulizer is still only about 40% of her best result. As a consequence she should be admitted to hospital for continued therapy.

Further information

Figure 2 is the adapted algorithm for the management of asthma in the Accident and Emergency department prepared by the British Thoracic Society. Figure 3 shows peak expiratory flow in normal adults.

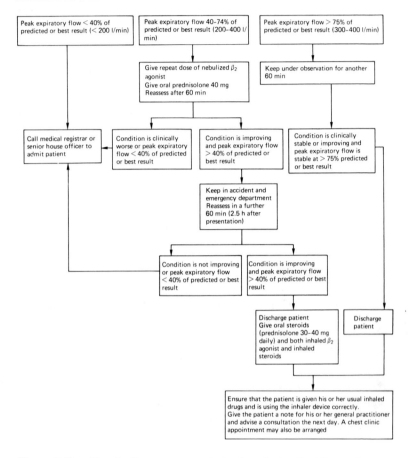

Figure 2 Algorithm for the management of asthma in the Accident and Emergency department. (Prepared by the British Thoracic Society)

References

British Thoracic Society (1990) Guidelines for treatment of asthma. *British Medical Journal,* **301**, 797, 799

Gregg, I. and Nunn, A. J. (1989) Peak expiratory flow in normal subjects. *British Medical Journal,* **298**, 1068–1070

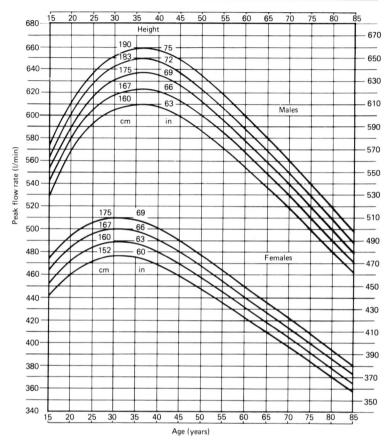

Figure 3 Peak expiratory flow in normal subjects. (From Gregg and Nunn (1989). With thanks to Clement Clark International)

Case 5

A 56-year-old man presented to the Accident and Emergency department with retrosternal chest pain which he described as a soreness. It had woken him from sleep at 02:00. The pain was initially severe and had made him sweat, lasted for 2 h, then had subsided sufficiently for him to fall back to sleep. He was woken again at 06:30 by the pain, which remained retrosternal and did not radiate. Nothing exacerbated the pain but belching did seem to improve it. In the past he had never suffered from exertional chest pain, but had recurrent indigestion after food and had had a hiatus hernia diagnosed following a barium meal, 10 years previously for which he took regular antacids. He was also taking enalapril for hypertension. He smoked 30 cigarettes/day and a brother had died of myocardial infarction aged 63.

On examination:

- He looked well, was pain free
- Obese
- Pulse 55/min, blood pressure 100/70 mmHg
- Chest clear, heart sounds normal
- Abdomen soft
- Rectal examination normal
- Chest radiograph normal
- Electrocardiogram very poor quality due to interference, but probably normal

Questions

1 What is the diagnosis?
2 What is your management?

Answers

1 The diagnosis lies between ischaemic cardiac and oesophageal pain. Retrosternal soreness that develops in a patient with a history of dyspepsia when recumbent in bed, which is eased by belching, may well be oseophageal in nature. However, it is very dangerous to attribute chest pain to an oesophageal cause (a diagnosis that cannot be confirmed in the Accident and Emergency department) unless there is overwhelming evidence of its existence, and no symptoms or risk factors that could implicate ischaemia. Retrosternal pain which wakes the patient from sleep as distinct from that which is exacerbated by lying flat should always be considered ischaemic in origin.

Emphasizing the history in the following fashion: 'A 56-year-old male developed retrosternal chest pain at rest, which lasted for 2 h and made him sweat. He was hypertensive, a smoker with a family history of ischaemic heart disease . . .' would suggest the pain is ischaemic in origin.

Often clinical examination is normal. However, in this patient further evidence of ischaemia is suggested by the bradycardia and the relative hypotension. It would be most unlikely that his blood pressure of 100/70 mmHg is solely due to his antihypertensive medication.

All patients presenting with similar symptoms, should be considered to have an ischaemic heart disease, and be referred for exclusion of a myocardial infarction.

2 Venous access should be established.
A good quality ECG should be obtained. Do not be tempted to make any management plans on an inadequate tracing.
Give the patient an aspirin 150 mg to chew.
Refer the patient for admission and exclusion of a myocardial infarction.

Outcome

A repeat ECG demonstrated ST elevation of 1 mm in lead II, and AVF which had been obscured by interference in the first tracing. He was treated with thrombolytic therapy and aspirin. Six hours later the ECG demonstrated a Q wave inferior infarct.

Further notes

The evaluation of a patient with possible ischaemic chest pain is a very common challenge to the clinician in Accident and Emergency. Misdiagnosis can be lethal. Aproximately 5% of patients who present acutely with a myocardial infarction, have their symptoms misinterpreted and are discharged.

The majority of patients presenting with acute myocardial infarction have typical symptoms with prolonged (>15 min) pain. The pain is centred in the anterior chest, between the nipples, described variously as 'tight', 'gripping', 'a dull ache' or 'constricting' and progressively becomes more severe. The pain may radiate to the neck, jaw, or down either or both arms. Nausea, vomiting and sweating commonly accompany the pain and the patient may complain of breathlessness. When a patient gives a history containing many of these features the diagnosis is obvious.

However, in some patients (most notably diabetics and the elderly) there may be only mild chest discomfort or no pain at all. In such cases the presenting complaint is usually of a non-specific nature such as 'feeling generally unwell' or 'sudden tiredness and lethargy'. Alternatively patients may present with syncope, or sudden deterioration in their normally well-controlled heart failure.

The diagnosis of ischaemic chest pain is most elusive, however, when patients fail to portray their symptoms in the recognized 'typical' fashion. The subjective appreciation of pain is very variable, and the words used to describe the episode may be more so. The experienced clinician will subconsciously run through a check list of points such as the site, nature and radiation of the pain, associated symptoms, risk factors for ischaemic heart disease etc. and form an impression of the patients symptoms, rather than discounting the episode because of an atypical description of the pain.

In an attempt to place patients in high or low risk categories for ischaemic disease based upon the description of the pain Lee *et al.* (1985) studied 596 patients (aged over 25) with acute chest pain as they presented as an emergency to hospital. Not surprisingly they found that myocardial infarctions were much more common in males age 40–70 than in any other age group. The percentage of patients who describe their chest pain as, a pressure, an ache, or as burning indigestion, who were ultimately shown to have had a myocardial infarction, were 24%, 13% and 23% respectively indicting that these descriptions of burning and indigestion were just as predictive of a myocardial infarction as the typical symptoms. Other words used to describe the pain of a myocardial infarction in these patients were 'a knot', 'suffocating' and 'bricks'.

When the pain was described as sharp and stabbing in quality, this qualitative description was much less predictive of myocardial infarction. Only 5% of 157 cases having a myocardial infarction.

In a similar review of patients with chest pain, Short (1981) in Aberdeen examined 456 episodes of spontaneous chest pain in 383 patients. He found that in patients, with no previous history of infarction or angina, who complained of pain that was affected by breathing, twisting or bending rarely had sustained a myocardial infarction. Similarly, for patients with a history of previous infarction or angina, if the site of the pain in the new episode was remote from the site of their previous event then this too was unlikely to be a new cardiac event.

With regard to associated symptoms there was a correlation between acute infarction and nausea (with or without vomiting) and sweating.

Short's study confirmed the fact that the majority of patients at presentation had no physical findings of note. However, when present, the findings of breathlessness and a tachycardia correlated with an acute ischaemic event.

Patients should be admitted on the strength of history, with or without supporting evidence from an electrocardiogram. From the data given above, guidelines as to which patients should be considered as high risk for an ischaemic event, and therefore admitted to hospital are:

1 Patients with a typical history of recent onset of angina, or infarction.
2 Patients (particularly males aged 40–70 years) with atypical pain, particularly when associated with nausea, sweating and breathlessness, and/or risk factors for ischaemic heart disease.
3 Patients with previous ischaemic episodes presenting with similar symptoms.

All such patients need admission to hospital, for serial ECGs and enzymes, and possibly exercise testing.

Cardiac risk factors

Major risk factors for ischaemic heart disease should always be sought. These include:

- known coronary artery disease
- hypertension
- smoking,
- family history,
- diabetes and hyperlipidaemia.

Remember patients without risk factors can have infarcts.

The role of the electrocardiogram

The ECG can be extremely helpful when evaluating patients with chest pain, however, it also can be very misleading. The ECG should always be examined in the light of the history.

Patients with ischaemic pain, usually have demonstrable changes on the ECG if it is recorded during the episode of pain. Likewise it is unusual for the ECG to be entirely 'normal' in the presence of an evolving full thickness myocardial infarction. I stress 'entirely normal' as minor or borderline changes should be treated with great suspicion, remembering that ECG changes may take several hours to become obviously abnormal.

If the ECG demonstrates ST elevation of even the slightest degree in any lead except AVR, V1, or V2, then the likelihood of acute infarction is great. The diagnosis of physiological high take off, rather than early ischaemia or pericarditis should be made retrospectively once an infarction has been excluded.

A normal ECG taken after the pain does not however exclude unstable angina, or coronary artery spasm, re-emphasizing the importance of the history rather than the ECG. If the history is suggestive of myocardial infarction or recent onset angina the patient should be admitted.

Comparison of the new ECG with previous ones can be very helpful when available. A significant difference between the two should be taken as an indication of further acute damage.

Practice points

1 Atypical chest pain poses a problem for all clinicians and most people have been caught out on more than one occasion. Ischaemic heart disease is very common and unfortunately not all describe typical symptoms. Any non-pleuritic pain felt in the anterior chest (between the nipples) in a patient with risk factors, which causes sweating and/or shortness of breath, should be considered ischaemic – in the absence of an obvious diagnosis.

2 A normal ECG does not exclude a myocardial infarction. The ECG is interpreted in the light of the history and examination, therefore never ask for a senior opinion on an ECG alone, but always on the patient.

3 Patients with undiagnosed ischaemic chest pain are commonly sent home. This is one of the commonest areas in which 'medical' medicolegal litigation occurs.

References

Lee, T. H. *et al.* (1985) Acute chest pain in the emergency room. *Archives of Internal Medicine,* **145**

Medical Defence Union, Personal communication

Short, D. (1981) Diagnosis of slight and subacute coronary attacks in the community. *British Heart Journal,* **45**, 299–310

Case 6

A 19-year-old man presented with pain in his left testicle which had started during a game of football. There had been no obvious trauma. The pain had increased in severity over 4 h, was exacerbated by walking, and relieved by lying down. He had been nauseated and had vomited once. Two weeks previously he had developed sudden pain in his left testicle during sexual intercourse, but this had spontaneously resolved within 10 min. He had noticed mild dysuria but no discharge over the past 10 days, and was otherwise well.

On examination:

- In pain
- Pyrexial 37.6°C
- Both testes were lying normally at the same level
- The left testis was too tender to touch and the overlying skin was red
- The epididymis of the right testicle was tender
- Rectal examination was normal, the prostate was non-tender
- No urethral discharge
- Urine clear

Questions

1 What is the diagnosis?
2 What is your management?

Answers

1 The differential diagnosis includes testicular torsion and acute epididymo-orchitis (Table 1). Torsion should be considered in any patient with an acutely swollen testicle. Testicular torsion most commonly occurs in adolescents and young adults, and it is the only diagnosis that should be entertained in a patient below the age of 30 years who presents with unilateral painful testis, until exploration has excluded it. Although much less common over the age of 30, it still occurs occasionally. By contrast, epididymo-orchitis most commonly occurs in patients over the age of 30 and is usually bilateral, although unilateral symptoms may predominate. However, the differentiation between the two is a common cause of diagnostic difficulty. The history may be helpful in distinguishing between the two conditions.

The pain in torsion usually starts abruptly, commonly during physical exercise or while asleep. The pain is severe and may be felt in the groin or abdomen, and the patient may vomit. Previous episodes of self-limiting pain may have been experienced. In contrast, the epididymo-orchitis is of insidious onset over days with gradually increasing scrotal discomfort, dysuria and occasionally discharge. The pain is not usually severe enough to make the patient vomit.

Clinically, however, both conditions can give rise to a tense, red, tender scrotal sac and a pyrexia. The torted testis may be higher than the normal side, have lost its cremasteric reflex, and lie in the horizontal plane (bell clapper testis). Examination of the normal testis often reveals a horizontal lie as the defect is usually bilateral. This is a useful diagnostic sign. The prostate is non-tender. Epididymitis represents ascending urethral infection (usually chlamydia in young men) which affects the epididymis and testicle via the prostate and vas deferens. It is frequently bilateral and the symptoms of prostatic infection are usually marked with urinary urgency, frequency and poor stream. Pyuria is a frequent finding as is a tender prostate.

Table 1 Differential diagnosis of testicular torsion and epididymo-orchitis

	Testicular torsion	*Epididymo-orchitis*
Onset of pain	Sudden	Gradual
Vomiting	Yes	No
Urinary symptoms	No	Yes
Pyuria	No	Yes
Tender prostate	No	Yes
Horizontal testis (bell clapper)	Yes	No
Horizontal normal testis	Yes	No
Loss of cremasteric reflex	Yes	No

2 This patient has had a short history of unilateral testicular pain, with vomiting, and irrespective of the other symptoms should be assumed to have torsion. Any patient below the age of 30 presenting with unilateral testicular pain should be referred to the surgeons for the exclusion of torsion, even if the diagnosis appears to be suggestive of infection. Patients above this age should be treated on their merits. All intermediate cases should be assumed to be torsion and referred for a surgical opinion. Doppler ultrasound and radionuclide scanning can be helpful in differentiating between the two conditions in this group, but should be requested by the surgeon.

The justification for this approach comes from the numerous case reports for patients all with symptoms and signs suggesting infection in whom the diagnosis was torsion. There is no sign which allows you confidently to exclude torsion on clinical examination and even previous orchidopexy does not exclude torsion.

Cautionary tale

A 32-year-old man presented with acute left testicular pain, and vomiting. Examination revealed a high, horizontal, tender testicle. Six years previously he had undergone a bilateral orchidopexy for torsion. Operation confirmed a torsion.

This approach may lead to as many as 30% of patients having a 'negative' exploration rate which many urologists feel is necessary not to miss a case.

Outcome

A necrotic testicle was removed at operation.

Practice point

Treat all unilaterally swollen, painful testicles as torsion.

Reference

Mitchell, J. P. chapter 51 in *Hamilton Bailey's Emergency Surgery* 11th edn. Wright, Bristol, 534

Case 7

A man was poked in the left eye by his 2-year-old son. He developed an acutely painful, watery eye, which was photophobic and had an intense foreign body sensation. Visual acuity 6/18 left, 6/6 right.

Questions

1 What is the diagnosis?

Five days later the symptoms were not improved, though the foreign body sensation had now resolved and the eye did not water as much. Clinical examination failed to demonstrate any corneal abnormality. Visual acuity 6/12 left, 6/6 right.
2 What is the diagnosis?

Answers

1 This is a typical history of corneal abrasion, and the condition is easy to diagnose. Instillation of fluorescein stains the abrasion green when viewed under blue light, highlighting the defect. Abrasions may interfere with vision leading to a reduction in visual acuity particularly if the abrasion is directly over the visual axis.

Management includes:

- exclusion of a corneal foreign body
- antibiotic ointment and drops
- eye pad
- review within 48 h
- give tetanus toxoid if necessary

Many abrasions will heal within 48 h, though some heal imperfectly leading to a recurrent erosion. Typically the patient gives a history of previous abrasion and then recurrent episodes of early morning pain and foreign body sensation. This is thought to occur as the imperfect epithelium is dislodged during REM sleep producing a recurrence of the abrasion.

2 The clinical examination excludes corneal abrasion as a continuing source of the symptoms. An anterior uveitis should be considered and the patient referred to the ophthalmology team.

Case 8

A woman of 75 years presented with a large subconjunctival haemorrhage of her left eye. There was no history of trauma. She was otherwise asymptomatic.
   Visual acuity (with glasses) 6/6 left, 6/9 right.

Question

What is your management?

Answer

Subconjunctival haemorrhage can occur spontaneously especially in the elderly. They may be precipitated by bouts of coughing, and are uncommonly the presenting features of anticoagulant overdose or blood dyscrasias.

In the absence of trauma, the patient can be reassured, and advised that it will take 2 weeks for the blood to resolve.

Recurrent spontaneous haemorrhages should be investigated with a full blood count and ESR.

When there is a history of trauma, the potential of a penetrating injury should be entertained. Is there a relevant history? The haemorrhage may be the only sign of a penetrating foreign body. Fractures of the orbital margin and the anterior cranial fossa are associated with subconjunctival haemorrhage, in these cases however, the history and examination make the diagnosis obvious with the haemorrhage being an incidental finding rather than the presenting complaint.

When there is a history suggestive of penetrating trauma, radiographs should be requested and the patient referred to the ophthalmology team.

Reference

Bron, A. J. and Davey, C. C. (1987) *The Unquiet Eye*. Glaxo Laboratories Ltd, Greenford

Case 9

A 6-year-old boy presented to the Accident and Emergency department with severe respiratory distress. He had been completely well until 20:00 the previous evening when he had developed a tickle in his throat and a cough. He had gone to bed but was unable to sleep because of a persistent coughing and some shortness of breath, his mother noted that he had a high temperature. At 01:00 because of increasing shortness of breath his mother took him to the local hospital. He was seen and assessed by the Accident and Emergency SHO, who made a diagnosis of asthma, prescribed nebulized salbutamol, felt that there had been significant improvement and discharged the patient home at 03:00.

At 08:00 the mother took the child to the local children's hospital, because of increasing respiratory distress. In the past the child had been well, there had been no previous attacks of wheezing or family history of asthma, eczema or allergy.

On examination:

- Pyrexial 40°C, drowsy and restless, well perfused
- Respiratory rate 48/min, pulse 155/min, blood pressure 100/70 mmHg
- No cyanosis
- Marked sternal and intercostal recession
- Using accessory muscles of respiration
- Inspiratory and expiratory stridor
- Very poor air entry
- No focal signs, chest signs
- No rash

Questions

1 What is your immediate management?
2 What is the differential diagnosis?
3 What lessons can be learnt from the actions of the Accident and Emergency SHO at the first hospital?

Answers

1 Immediate management

This child has severe respiratory distress which could prove to be fatal if not relieved immediately.

- Reassure mother and child
- Sit the child up. Lying flat may increase upper airway obstruction
- Give high concentration of oxygen via mask. If the child will not tolerate wearing the mask, mother should hold it as close as possible to the face without disturbing the child
- Call for senior help. The consultant in Accident and Emergency, senior anaesthetist, paediatrician, and ENT surgeon should all be called immediately
- Nebulized adrenaline (0.5–1 mg) may be helpful while waiting for the anaesthetist. (Heliox is an alternative to oxygen)
- Ensure that all the equipment for emergency airway support is at hand namely:
  bag and mask connected to the oxygen support;
  intubation equipment with the right size tube;
  a cannula for needle cricothyroidotomy;
  emergency tracheostomy set

(If in doubt about the endotracheal tube size approximate by preparing a tube whose internal diameter, is the same as the diameter of the child's little finger. Or by using the formula of age/4 + 4.5 which is a reliable guide for the size of endotracheal tubes necessary in children but less so for infants.)

Do not

- Attempt to visualize the throat
- Take blood
- Set up a drip
- Request radiographs or do anything else that may upset the child

Management

This child should be intubated by a skilled anaesthetist in theatre, in the presence of an ENT surgeon, who is available to perform an emergency tracheostomy if required.

The child should be slowly anaesthetized in a calm environment using inhalational anaesthesia to a level where the larynx can be directly visualized. If the obstruction is supraglottic as in epiglottitis, and intubation is impossible, a tracheostomy should be performed. Once intubated, the airway is secure, and now venous access should be established and further investigation and treatment can be undertaken.

2 Differential diagnosis

The commonest cause of acute stridor in infants is the viral condition of laryngotracheobronchitis, commonly called croup. However any child presenting with the triad of stridor, toxaemia and respiratory embarrassment should be considered to have acute epiglottitis. Below are the clinical features of the conditions which may give rise to acute stridor.

Laryngotracheobronchitis

It is usually caused by the parainfluenza virus, or less commonly by the respiratory syncytial virus, or rhinovirus, and has a peak incidence during the second year of life. The typical history is one of a preceding coryzal illness for 1–2 days prior to the development of a barking cough, hoarseness and then stridor. The stridor is aggravated by crying and can be absent at rest. Most children do not experience serious respiratory difficulty, but a few will develop tachypnoea associated with marked intercostal recession. In severe cases hypoxia, restlessness, exhaustion and cyanosis develop and about 1–2% of children admitted to hospital with this condition will need intubation and ventilation. Features of systemic upset are usually absent even in these children, that is the child is not toxic.

Typically, children with croup present with their parents in the early hours of the morning as this is when symptoms are usually worse. Both parents and child are agitated which exacerbates the symptoms. Gentle handling and careful observation in hospital are necessary.

Acute epiglottitis

This rapidly progressive disease accounts for less than 10% of all hospital admissions for acute stridor. It usually affects children aged 2–7 years, but has been described in adults. It is nearly always caused by *Haemophilus influenzae* type B which, in addition to causing gross oedema of the epiglottis, gives rise to a ring of inflamed oedematous tissue surrounding the supraglottic laryngeal space. In contrast to acute laryngotracheobronchitis the onset is rapid, over hours not days, and being a septicaemic illness the child looks acutely unwell from the outset. The child, previously well, quickly becomes toxic, cyanosed, and drools. Stridor develops with evidence of severe respiratory embarrassment and, in contrast to croup, cough is not a prominent symptom.

Bacterial tracheitis (pseudomembranous croup)

This condition is uncommon and presents in a similar way to epiglottitis with a toxic child in respiratory distress. A bacterial inflammation of the trachea produces a subglottic obstruction by giving rise to mucopus and sloughed epithelium. *Staphylococcus aureus* has been the predominant organism, and it usually affects children over the age of 5 years. There is usually a very short prodromal illness before fever, toxicity and respiratory distress develop.

Less common conditions

Other conditions such as an inhaled foreign body, and the uncommon angioneurotic oedema might both present with the sudden onset of stridor and respiratory embarrassment. The history of an inhaled foreign body is that of acute stridor developing in a previously well apyrexial infant. There might be a history of coughing at the outset when the foreign body is inhaled. Angioneurotic oedema causes swelling of the larynx and stridor as a consequence. Evidence of oedema elsewhere, i.e. tongue, face and pharynx, and urticaria, erythema or a rash may be present. There may be a family history, or a history of drug ingestion, e.g. aspirin, but often there is no obvious precipitating cause.

3 Lessons learnt

Upper airway obstruction can mimic asthma, as inspiratory and expiratory stridor might be mistaken for wheeze. However, it is very unwise to treat and discharge a child in the middle of the night, when the presenting illness was one of respiratory difficulty and a fever. All such patients and all asthmatics should be admitted and observed overnight at the very least.

Any child brought to the department during the night, indicates a high degree of concern on behalf of the guardian, whether well-founded or not, and I believe serious consideration should be given to admitting all such children.

Outcome

In this child the supraglottic region was normal, and intubation was performed with partial relief of the respiratory distress. Suction was performed from the trachea revealing frank mucopus which grew *Staphylococcus aureus*. A diagnosis of bacterial tracheitis was made. Antibiotics were commenced and the child made an uneventful recovery.

Reference

Browning G. G. (1987) *Updated ENT*. 2nd edn. Butterworths, Guildford

Case 10

A 22-year-old woman ate fish for lunch. She developed a sharp pricking sensation in her throat during the meal, which then persisted for 12 h. She had been able to swallow since, though each time she did so, she was aware of the sensation. She indicated the site of the sensation as being on the right side of her neck by the angle of the jaw.

Question

What is your management?

Answer

After ingestion the majority of fish bones become lodged in the oropharynx. Here they seem to have a predilection for the base of the tongue and the tonsillar fossa. Other less common places for fish bones to lodge are the piriformis fossae or upper oesophagus.

Patients commonly present with a feeling of something stuck in their throat after eating fish or, less commonly, chicken and meat.

The most important rule to remember when seeing these patients is to assume that a foreign body is present until proved otherwise.

Management

1 *History*: What has been ingested – fish, chicken? How long ago? What are the symptoms? Has the patient been able to swallow since? Commonly the answer to this last question is yes, patients with total dysphagia usually present immediately spitting up saliva. Can they lateralize the foreign body? If they can it suggests the bone is above the cricopharyngeus, in the hypopharynx, or oropharynx.

2 *Examination*: The neck should be examined for tenderness, masses or surgical emphysema. With the aid of a good light source, the mouth and pharynx should be examined.

The tonsillar fossa, base of tongue and posterior pharyngeal wall should be closely inspected. Strands of saliva are commonly mistaken for fish bones. A mirror will aid in examining the tonsil and the base of the tongue from a different angle, if no bone is obvious. If the patient finds it difficult to tolerate the mirror, the posterior pharyngeal wall should be anaesthetized. If no foreign body is seen then attempt to visualize the larynx. Indirect laryngoscopy is one of the most difficult clinical examinations to perform effectively. For the inexperienced the cords may be only glimpsed fleetingly. One should be looking for pooling of saliva, which may be the only visible indication of a foreign body. Foreign bodies in the region of the larynx need expert removal.

Soft tissue radiography

When no foreign body is seen, a lateral soft tissue radiograph of the neck should be requested. An adequate film is one which demonstrates all seven cervical vertebra. The cricopharyngeus is at the level of the sixth cervical vertebra and this area needs to be scrutinized, as it is the commonest place for an oesophageal foreign body to lodge. The actual foreign body may not be visible, particularly given the fact that the fish most commonly eaten in this country, mackerel, trout, salmon etc. have poorly radiopaque bones.

Indirect evidence of a foreign body should be sought. These signs include soft tissue swelling, gas in the soft tissues and air in the upper oesophagus. Be aware that these signs may take several hours to become obvious. Calcification in the thyroid cartilage and hyoid can make interpretation of these films difficult.

A normal radiograph is helpful, but it is not a substitute for a thorough clinical examination.

If no foreign body is seen then the following patients should be referred to the duty ENT surgeon.

1 All patients with total dysphagia.
2 All patients in whom clinical examination has been inadequate due to inexperience of the observer, or poor patient compliance.
3 All patients with positive findings on the radiograph.

Patients in whom no foreign body is seen after adequate examination, and a normal radiograph may be discharged. They should be reviewed within 48 h in the ENT outpatients if symptoms persist.

Outcome

A fish bone was found at the base of the patient's left tonsil. This was removed, with relief of the symptoms. She was discharged.

Further notes

Knight and Lesser (1989) studied all patients complaining of a sharp sensation in the throat after eating fish who presented to their department in one year. They collected 71 patients, 15 (21%) were found to have a fish bone, which was removed, (14 on initial examination, one needing endoscopy). The remaining 56 (79%) had no obvious foreign body and were discharged, being asked to return in 48 h to the ENT clinic if their symptoms persisted. Fifteen patients did so, but no further foreign bodies were found. Four patients were still symptomatic at 2 weeks, and all had a negative endoscopy. Two of this group continued to be symptomatic at 3 months and, despite extensive investigation, no foreign body was found. The authors concluded that the majority of patients with symptoms of a lodged foreign body after eating fish had been scratched by the bone, the bone having passed on at the time of presentation. There are however numerous case reports of undetected bones of various sorts giving rise to fatal mediastinitis from oesophageal perforation. Therefore, there is no substitute for complete clinical examination. If your examination has been incomplete ask advice from your consultant or the duty ENT surgeon.

Reference

Knight, L. C. and Lesser, T. H. J. (1989) Fish bones in the throat. *Archives of Emergency Medicine*, **6**, 13–16

Case 11

A 21-year-old man had a lucky escape when the warehouse he was working in caught fire. He was stocktaking in the office at the rear of the warehouse when he first smelled smoke. He opened the office door to find the whole warehouse full of smoke. The only means of escape was through the warehouse itself.

He was found by the ambulance men, drowsy, confused and rambling by the fire exit. The fire that produced the smoke was in the opposite corner of the warehouse, and although he was covered in soot, he did not appear to have been burnt.

With the administration of oxygen in the ambulance his condition improved, and by the time he arrived at the Accident and Emergency department he was fully awake and orientated and able to give a clear history of the event.

He now complained of a cough, sore throat, chest tightness and shortness of breath. There was no serious past medical history of note. In particular he was not asthmatic and did not smoke.

On examination:
- Distressed
- Coughing
- Covered in soot, and particles of soot in his mouth, though no obvious oedema or burns of the mouth or pharynx
- Hoarse voice
- Respiratory rate 18/min
- No stridor
- Widespread wheeze throughout the chest
- Heart sounds normal
- No cutaneous burn
- The remainder of the examination is normal

Questions

1 What are the potential problems associated with the inhalation of smoke?
2 How do you make the clinical diagnosis of smoke inhalation?
3 What is your immediate management of this patient?
4 What are the clinical features of carbon monoxide poisoning, and its treatment?

Answers

1 Significant problems

Significant inhalation injury is a common cause of death in patients with extensive burns, though patients with isolated smoke inhalation usually survive. It is however a common cause of morbidity and needs to be recognized and treated promptly.

The inhalation of smoke gives rise to two major problems:

systemic poisoning
injury to the respiratory tract.

Systemic poisoning: noxious substances in smoke are absorbed and act as cellular poisons. The most ubiquitous of these is carbon monoxide, although others such as hydrogen cyanide and sulphide and carbon dioxide are also commonly present.

Carbon monoxide not only is capable of direct cellular damage, but also leads to cellular hypoxia by forming carboxyhaemoglobin and shifting the oxyhaemoglobin curve to the left.

Carboxyhaemoglobin levels should always be estimated in patients with suspected inhalational injury. High levels would indicate significant inhalation though normal levels, especially if taken some hours after the exposure do not exclude significant tissue toxicity.

Inhalational injury to the respiratory tract: direct thermal damage accounts for a limited percentage of the respiratory problems and is usually confined to the upper airways due to efficient heat-exchanging tissues of the nose, pharynx and larynx. On occasion, however, hot gases may cause damage to the lower airways and the lung parenchyma.

Irritants contained in the smoke give rise to much of the airways damage, either by direct chemical damage, or by damaging the normally protective mechanisms such as the mucociliary escalator. Certain irritants such as sulphur dioxide in particular are likely to give rise to bronchospasm.

2 Clinical diagnosis of smoke inhalation

A clinical diagnosis of inhalational injury can be assumed if more than two of the following risk factors are present:

- A history of exposure to smoke in a confined space
- A history of altered consciousness or confusion at any time since the exposure
- Evidence of perioral burns – to lips, mouth, pharynx or singed nostril hairs
- i Symptoms of mucous membrane irritation with watery eyes, sore throat
  ii Cough and symptoms of respiratory irritation with breathlessness, tight chest, wheezing or a sense of choking or suffocation
- Clinical signs of respiratory involvement such as:
  i laboured breathing with increased respiratory rate
  ii stridor
  iii wheeze
- Hoarseness or loss of voice

- The production of carbonaceous spatium or soot deposits in the mouth or pharynx

3 Management

This man presents with a history of prolonged exposure to smoke in an enclosed environment, altered consciousness and examination finds him to be wheezy, have a hoarse voice and have soot particles in his mouth. A confident diagnosis of smoke inhalation can be made.

Immediate management consists of:

- 60% oxygen given by Venturi mask.
- Nebulized salbutamol 5 mg for wheeze.
- Measure arterial blood gases and the carboxyhaemoglobin level (see below).
- Inform the anaesthetist and arrange admission to a high dependency area/intensive care. A chest radiograph can be performed once stabilized in a high dependency area, as there are no early changes associated with smoke inhalation. However, it is useful as a base line investigation and to demonstrate pre-existing disease.

Intubation and ventilation with 100% oxygen is necessary for any patient with altered consciousness or coma on arrival who may have smoke inhalation. Elective intubation should be considered in all patients with the potential for upper airway obstruction, such as intraoral burns or pharyngeal oedema, before stridor and respiratory embarrassment develop. Intubation and ventilation are mandatory if the patient cannot tolerate the face mask or maintain a clear airway.

Fibreoptic bronchoscopy is used increasingly frequently to assesss the upper, and lower airway for evidence of respiratory tract damage. Frank ulceration and bleeding, carbon particles and chemical burn coagulum would all be direct evidence of smoke inhalation.

Note on arterial blood gases

In the presence of carbon monoxide poisoning P_aO_2 levels may be spuriously high. This is because a conventional blood gas analyser calculates the P_aO_2 on the assumption that only normal haemoglobin is present. If carboxyhaemoglobin is present in high quantities, as it is not available for O_2 binding, the P_aO_2 can be unrepresentative. (The same is true for oximetry.)

Outcome

This man was given 60% oxygen and a salbutamol nebulizer. The anaesthetist felt that there was no risk of imminent upper airway obstruction. His carboxyhaemoglobin level was 23% and he was referred to the local hyperbaric unit.

4 Clinical features of carbon monoxide poisoning and treatment

Carbon monoxide poisoning should always be considered when there has been exposure to smoke. In other circumstances however it is commonly overlooked.

Carbon monoxide is produced by car exhausts, poorly ventilated heating systems and inhaled fumes from paint stripper (via the liver).

Symptoms of poisoning are often non-specific and include weakness, nausea, vomiting, headache, lethargy and dyspnoea. Clinical signs are equally non-specific and usually attributed to another cause. These include altered consciousness, coma, confusion, hyperflexia and cardiac instability and arrhythmias. The so-called typical 'cherry red' skin colour is rarely seen except in fatalities.

If recognized or suspected, the carboxyhaemoglobin level should be estimated. Levels below 5% are considered normal; however, levels as high as 9% may be found in smokers.

Treatment consists of 100% oxygen with a tight-fitting mask, and the consideration of hyperbaric oxygen treatment.

The indications for hyperbaric treatment are:

- conscious patient with carboxyhaemoglobin > 20% at any time
- neurological symptoms other than headache at any time, or neurological signs
- pregnancy
- cardiac ischaemia or arrhythmias

Relevant contraindications to hyperbaric therapy in a monoplace (one man) chamber:

- patients who are ventilated or who are not able to maintain an airway due to altered consciousness
- life-threatening cardiac instability
- asthma

For your local/nearest unit contact Plymouth, Diving Diseases Research Centre, tel: 0752 408093.

Cautionary tale
A 44-year-old man was found in a coma at home by his wife on her return from a business trip. The only relevant history was that in the last week he had been complaining of 'flu-like' symptoms.

In hospital the cause of the illness was not obvious. Carbon monoxide poisoning was only suspectd when the next day his wife returned to hospital having spent the night at home, complaining of a headache, and 'flu-like' symptoms.

The insidious nature of carbon monoxide poisoning is demonstrated well by the case report in *The British Medical Journal* (1990, **301**, 997) by Crawford *et al.*

Acknowledgement

Thanks to Dr M Hamilton-Farrell, Consultant in Charge of the Hyperbaric Unit, Whipps Cross Hospital, London

Case 12

A 34-year-old man presented to Accident and Emergency with an increasingly severe headache. Four weeks previously he had been admitted to hospital after falling from a horse sustaining a head injury. He had lost consciousness for about 15 min. He could not recall any event that occurred immediately after the injury, such as how he came to be in hospital, but did remember having had his skull radiographed and events thereafter. His post-traumatic amnesia was calculated to be about one hour. After overnight observation he was allowed home, without follow-up, and was informed that he had not fractured his skull.

His headache had been present in hospital, and had slowly increased in severity since that time. Nothing he did relieved the headache, but was aware that many different things made it worse such as walking, talking and coughing. His sleep had been disturbed, and he often woke in the early morning at 05–06:00 unable to return to sleep. There were other symptoms of lethargy, lack of interest and concentration, and lightheadedness every time he stood up. He had lost his appetite, which he attributed to the continual nausea that he experienced, and over the last 10 days he had vomited several times a day when he tried to eat.

This was the fourth Accident and Emergency department that he had been to in the past 2 weeks because as he said, 'I know that there is something wrong inside my head'.

On examination:

- Apyrexial, flat affect, spent most of the consultation with his eye closed Glasgow coma score 15
- Higher cerebral function save concentration was normal. (He was obviously irritated by many of the questions)
- Cranial nerves intact, no nystagmus
- Visual fields, visual acuity and fundi normal
- No meningism
- Ears normal
- There were no focal neurological signs
- Gait and balance normal

- Scalp tender to touch, but no signs of injury
- Blood pressure 130/80 mmHg, pulse 80/min regular
- The rest of the physical examination was normal

Question

What diagnosis should you consider?

Answer

The diagnoses which should be considered are the post-concussional syndrome and a subdural collection.

Many patients present to Accident and Emergency with persisting symptoms of a head injury. The symptoms often appear disproportionately severe by comparison with the initial insult. The severity of a head injury can be graded according to the length of the post-traumatic amnesia.

<5 mins	very mild
<1 h	mild
1–24 h	moderate
1–7 days	severe
>7 days	very severe

It has been recognized that the severity of the post-traumatic symptoms depends more upon the individual than the severity of injury. This compounded with the fact that undoubtedly some patients' symptoms improved dramatically on being awarded compensation has led some people to suggest that the symptoms have a functional basis. But the similarity of the type of symptoms experienced by patients, together with the fact that it has been shown that as little as 5 min of unconsciousness can be associated with diffuse axonal damage, would suggest an organic basis.

The term post-concussional syndrome has been used to describe a host of post head-injury symptoms. Commonly recognized symptoms include headache, dizziness or lightheadedness, symptoms of anxiety or depression, impairment of concentration and memory, irritability, fatigue and photophobia. The symptoms usually start at the end of the post-traumatic amnesia and usually resolve over the ensuing weeks or months. Premature return to work, or other stressful environments can exacerbate symptoms. When there is a delay in onset of the symptoms after injury of several weeks the symptoms are more likely to have a functional basis.

Sympathetic handling at the time of the acute injury, and full written explanation of the common symptoms should be given to the patients along with the head injury warning instructions at the time of discharge in an attempt to aid recovery.

In addition to the post-concussional syndrome, symptoms from cranial nerve damage may also cause continuing symptoms. The commonest nerves to be damaged are the first, giving rise to anosmia, which can be found in up to 10% of all head injuries, and damage to the eighth nerve as it enters the internal auditory meatus. Lesions to both of these nerves are common in patients without skull fractures and are due to stretching or tearing of the nerves when there is sudden movement of the intracranial contents at the time of injury. Anosmia is a rare complaint but the vertigo, tinnitus and hearing loss associated with eighth nerve damage are usually noticed early in the recovery phase. The loss of balance can be a serious hindrance to speedy recovery.

This patient has many of the symptoms of the post-concussional syndrome and this is the most likely diagnosis. However, it is important to identify those patients whose symptoms and/or signs suggest the presence of an intercranial collection. Neurosurgical advice should be sought for the following:

1 Fluctuating level of consciousness
2 Increasing headache with or without persisting vomiting
3 Change in personality or confusion
4 Focal neurological signs
5 Cerebrospinal fluid leak
6 True diplopia
7 Epileptic fit

1 Fluctuating level of consciousness

A history of periods of excessive drowsiness during the day is of particular significance, and the chances of finding a focal collection are high. Patients who have very disturbed sleep at night, and then snooze during the day, as this man, are naturally tired and not excessively drowsy.

Remember A history of fluctuating consciousness is the cardinal symptom in a patient with a chronic subdural haematoma.

2 Increasingly severe headache (not relieved by simple analgesia), particularly when associated with persistent vomiting

Headache is a very common sequela of head injury (usually due to a small quantity of blood in the subarachnoid space), although the severity and duration are variable. Patients should be advised to lie flat and rest for a number of days until the headache improves and then are allowed up. If the headache returns then they should again return to the recumbent position. The trend however is a slow improvement in the headache and therefore an increasingly severe headache, especially one that is worse in the morning is an ominous symptom. Persistent vomiting on a daily basis is another significant symptom.

3 Change in personality or confusion

Subtle changes in a patient's personality or a history of confusion readily noticed by close friends and relatives, and perhaps not so obvious to medical personnel may be due to diffuse axonal damage, but when present shortly after a head injury may be the only sign of a focal lesion.

4 Focal neurological signs

In general these are late signs and are usually associated with altered consciousness. The presence of a hemiparesis, pupil inequality, and papilloedema would obviously merit further investigation. These signs – particularly early papilloedema – may be very subtle, and its absence is of no particular importance.

5 Cerebrospinal fluid leak

Other symptoms which should not be overlooked are those associated with a dural tear and leak of CSF. Either otorrhoea or rhinorrhoea may have been noticed by the patients in the days following a head injury, and a history of both should be specifically enquired about. Otorrhoea is usually transient and often missed, and rhinorrhoea may be misinterpreted as being either a cold or non-specific rhinitis (see Cautionary tale p. 41).

6 Double vision

True diplopia should always be taken seriously. When a patient complains of being able to see two distinct images, and one of the images disappears on closing one eye, this is true diplopia. True diplopia in ambulant patients after head injury appears uncommon, and if present is due to orbital injury rather than a focal intercranial lesion, though fourth nerve palsy and other cranial nerve injuries are well documented.

Much more commonly however, patients report episodes of blurred vision or 'ghosting' in which one image slightly overlaps the other. Unlike true diplopia 'ghosting' persists when one eye is closed, and is due to uncorrected errors of refraction or mild lens opacities. Why patients appear particularly prone to be aware of this after a head injury is not clear.

7 Epileptic fit

The history of an epileptiform seizure after a head injury, in a patient not known to have fits would be an indication for a CT scan. Both early epilepsy (within one week of the head injury) and late epilepsy are most common in patients after a severe head injury (post-traumatic amnesia greater than 24 h) and those with either a depressed skull fracture or intracranial haematoma. For patients known to be epileptic, a sudden change in fit frequency would be a similar clinical indication for further investigation.

Outcome

This man's symptoms were discussed with the neurosurgeons. Although it was felt that the post-concussional syndrome was the most likely diagnosis, the history of persisting headache and vomiting gave rise to concern. A CT scan was normal. The patient was reassured and advised that his symptoms would improve, and he was referred back to his general practitioner for further follow up.

Cautionary tales
1 A young woman presented with a headache, dizziness, anorexia, and altered sleep pattern 4 days after a head injury. She had fallen backwards off a small wall and hit the back of her head on the ground. There had been no loss of consciousness. One hour post injury she had a nose bleed for about 30 min which stopped spontaneously. Since that time she had an intermittently runny nose, and a salty taste (CSF) at the back of her throat. She was unconcerned by this and did not complain of it. She was discharged home with the diagnosis of the post-concussional syndrome. A week later she was readmitted with meningitis.
2 A 68-year-old man with chronic lymphocytic leukaemia fell onto his face when drunk 8 days previously, but he was unsure whether he had lost consciousness. He presented because his nose was obviously deformed. He gave a history that for the first 2 days his nose had bled, but this had settled. For the last 2 days he had been troubled by a constant clear discharge from both nostrils, which he volunteered became much more troublesome during micturition. A small drop of fluid was obtained by getting him to put his head between his legs and straining. It was found positive for glucose when tested with a BM stix confirming it as CSF. He was admitted to hospital, treated prophylactically with antibiotics and the rhinorrhoea settled spontaneously.

Detection of CSF leak

1 If clear discharge – check with BM stix. CSF positive for glucose.
2 If blood-stained discharge – perform ring test – place a drop of fluid on filter paper, which will allow blood and CSF to separate into two distinct rings.

Further notes on subdural haematoma

In a review of 389 cases of subdural haematomata, McKissock (1960) arbitrarily defined 'acute' as those presenting within 3 days of injury, 'subacute' as those presenting within 4–20 days, and 'chronic' those presenting 21 days and after.

The commonest symptoms, experienced by these patients, and the clinical signs found at presentation in all three groups are shown below:

	Acute (82 cases) (%)	Subacute (91 cases) (%)	Chronic (216 cases) (%)
Alteration in consciousness	100	88	47
Headache	11	52	81
Confusion	12	42	38
Vomiting	25	31	30
Focal signs			
motor signs	44	37	41
pupil inequality	57	27	20
papilloedema	1	15	22
Epilepsy	6	3	9

Without a history of head injury, patients presenting with the above symptoms are often misdiagnosed as having cerebrovascular disease, brain tumours or psychiatric disease. Cameron (1978) reviewed 114 cases of chronic subdural haematoma and could only identify an obvious head injury in 55%, and pointed to the high rate of misdiagnosis in the absence of such an injury.

He felt that the majority of these 114 cases, presented with one of three groups of symptoms: (a) hemiparesis; (b) personality or intellectual change; (c) features of raised intracranial pressure; and that a chronic subdural haematoma should be included in the differential diagnosis of any patient presenting with such symptoms.

Practice points

1 Post-concussional symptoms are very common after head injury, and patients should be told not only to rest in bed until their headache settles but also be given written instructions about common associated symptoms they may experience.
2 A full history and thorough examination is necessary to elicit sinister symptoms and signs which may be indicative of an intercranial haematoma.
3 Patients with suggestive symptoms and signs should be considered for neurosurgical evaluation and CT.
4 Where post-concussional symptoms persist, follow-up by the patient's general practitioner is most appropriate and ensures that the patient can be referred back for further treatment if necessary.

References

Cameron, M. (1978) Chronic subdural haematoma: a review of 114 cases. *Journal of Neurology, Neurosurgery, and Psychiatry*, **41**, 834–839
McKissock, W. (1960) Subdural haematoma: a review of 389 cases. *Lancet*, **i**, 1365–1369

Case 13

A 3-year-old female child was brought by her mother with a 10-day history of unilateral nasal discharge, and what she described as very bad breath. She admitted that the smell had been so bad that she was reluctant to cuddle the child. She described the discharge as being green, tenacious, and occasionally blood-stained. There had been no other symptoms, or serious past medical history.

Questions

1 What is the likely diagnosis?
2 What is the management?

Answers

1 Diagnosis

The diagnosis is a retained foreign body in the nose. The history is typical of an impacted foreign body and the foul smell is due to superadded infection. The foreign body usually lies on the nasal floor at the level of the inferior turbinate.

2 Management

With a history of a chronically impacted foreign body up the nose, refer the child to the duty ENT surgeons. Mucosal oedema, discharge and pain will all decrease the chances of successful removal. You may be successful when the foreign body has only been retained for several hours.

Management of retained foreign bodies in children is always difficult whether they are in the nose or ear. The child usually only allows you one attempt, so the initial assessment about the feasibility of removal is all important.

The essential questions to ask oneself before removing a foreign body whether in the nose, or the ear in a child are first, 'Is there a good chance I can remove this foreign body in one go?' and second, 'Can I do this without causing any further damage?' e.g. perforating the ear drum. If you are unsure about either question refer the child before attempting removal.

It is not uncommon for the drum to be perforated or ossicles to be removed by the inexperienced.

If attempting to remove the foreign body, explain the procedure fully to the guardian and obtain her cooperation.

The following are essential for success:

- Secure handling of the child. With the aid of a blanket, the guardian and an experienced nurse the child should be immobilized in a firm but kind manner.
- A good light source.
- Correct instruments for removal, e.g. ear syringe – the majority of foreign bodies in the ear can be removed by syringing including insects; Tilley's forceps or hook; eustachian catheter – a useful non-traumatic instrument for beads in the nose.
- A steady hand, and a degree of confidence (never over confidence).

Urgency of removal

Nose: fairly urgent. Same day because of possibility of inhalation. Button batteries should be removed immediately as they can produce extensive corrosive damage.
Ear: next outpatients, provided no vertigo or acute pain.

If unsuccessful, refer to the ENT surgeons. Many such foreign bodies are removed under a general anaesthetic.

Outcome

This child had an impacted piece of sponge up her left nostril which was removed under a general anaesthetic.

Reference

Ludman, H. (1988) *ABC of Ear, Nose and Throat*. BMJ Publications, London

Case 14

A 70-year-old man from New Zealand was enjoying a holiday in Europe when one day he began to feel unwell. As the day progressed he became increasingly aware of rapid regular palpitations but denied chest pain or shortness of breath. As he often had palpitations he ignored them. While walking in the street however he tripped over, and injured his wrist, and so presented to the Accident and Emergency department. While being triaged the nurse assessed his radial pulse and discovered that he had a tachycardia of 150/min. She immediately placed him on a couch and attached him to a monitor and recorded his blood pressure. While an ECG was being performed the senior house officer in Accident and Emergency obtained the following history. He had been well recently save for an attack of severe indigestion 2 days previously which had lasted for 3 h and left him feeling rather tired. This had responded to some white medicine and he had not had the pain since. In the past, aged 46 years he had an inferior myocardial infarction and at the age of 52 a testicle was removed because of a 'growth'. He had been a life-long smoker, he drank alcohol regularly. He was not on any regular medication.

On examination:

- He looked well
- Apyrexial
- He was warm, and well perfused, respiratory rate 18/min; pulse 150/min; blood pressure 170/100 mmHg
- Chest was clear, no evidence of heart failure
- His abdomen was soft
- Right wrist – clinical Colles' fracture
- The rest of the examination was normal
- Monitor: revealed a broad complex tachycardia
- The ECG is shown in Figure 4

Questions

1 What is the diagnosis?
2 What is your immediate management?

Answers

1 Diagnosis

The ECG diagnosis is ventricular tachycardia. The electrocardiogram demonstrates a broad complex tachycardia. The possible diagnosis includes:

a Ventricular tachycardia
b Supraventricular tachycardia with pre-existing bundle branch block. That is, the patient normally has either left or right bundle branch block when in sinus rhythm
c Supraventricular tachycardia with rate-related bundle branch block (that is phasic aberrant conduction). This is usually (80%) right bundle branch block which tends to repolarize more slowly than the left bundle.

The diagnosis of ventricular tachycardia can be difficult. There are two common misconceptions associated with the diagnosis of ventricular tachycardia. These are that, ventricular tachycardia is irregular, and that patients with sustained ventricular tachycardia are always haemodynamically compromised. Neither of these two statements is correct. In the absence of fusion or captured beats, ventricular tachycardia is regular,

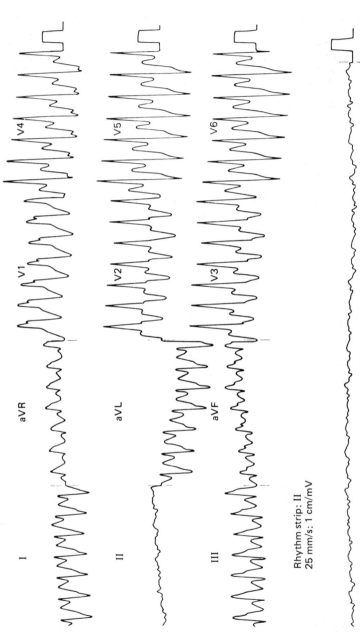

Rhythm strip: II
25 mm/s; 1 cm/mV

Figure 4 ECG from patient

and it does not always lead to a haemodynamic disturbance. The importance of differentiating between ventricular tachycardia and supraventricular tachycardia is that the treatment and prognosis differ with each group. The inappropriate treatment of a ventricular tachycardia with intravenous verapamil often leads to catastrophic haemodynamic deterioration, and left untreated ventricular tachycardia may deteriorate into ventricular fibrillation. Prompt diagnosis and appropriate treatment are necessary.

History and examination

The history might give some indication as to the origin of broad complex tachycardia. Baerman *et al.* (1987) evaluated factors in the history, and found that the following points had a high predictive value for ventricular tachycardia:

- age greater than 35 years – predictive value 85%
- history of congestive cardiac failure – predictive value 100%
- history of myocardial infarction – predictive value 98%
- history of recent angina – predictive value 100%

None of the historical factors was strongly predictive for supraventricular tachycardia. The best was an age of 35 years or less, which had a predictive value of 70%. Physical examination may demonstrate the presence of atrioventricular (AV) dissociation. Irregular canon waves may be visible at the neck and variable intensity of the first heart sounds might be found on auscultation and these are helpful signs. However, no definite conclusions can be drawn from the absence of these signs, as up to 30% of patients with ventricular tachycardia may have no AV dissociation.

Electrocardiogram

The examination of the ECG allows differentiation between a supraventricular and a ventricular origin in the majority of cases.

ECG features which favour a ventricular origin

i *Electrocardiographic evidence of AV dissociation*: if there is obvious evidence of AV dissociation with 'P' waves marching through the 'QRS' complexes, then the origin is likely to be ventricular. However, finding a one-to-one relationship between 'P' waves and the 'QRS' complexes although favours a supraventricular origin also occurs in up to 30% of patients with ventricular tachycardia.

ii *Broad complexes*: the broader the 'QRS' complex the more likely the arrhythmia is ventricular in origin. If the 'QRS' complexes have a duration of more than 0.14 s (over 3.5 small squares) it is unlikely to be supraventricular in origin.

iii *Fusion and captured beats*: both fusion and captured beats have a different morphology than the other beats in the tachycardia and are therefore easily recognized. Fusion beats represent the waveform produced when the ventricle is depolarized from two different sources. One beat arises in the atrium and captures the ventricle and another beat arises in the ventricular myocardium. The summation of both these waveforms gives rise to a fusion beat. A captured beat on the other hand is produced when there is antegrade capture of the ventricles by a sinus beat which captures the ventricle before the expected tachycardia 'QRS'. The presence of either a fusion or captured beat is indicative of a ventricular origin.

iv *Bizarre frontal plane axis*: the presence of left axis deviation (more than 30°) especially in the presence of right bundle branch block, or finding a positive complex in lead AVR are both suggestive of ventricular tachycardia.

v *Concordance*: concordance is said to occur when the 'QRS' complexes in the chest leads are either all positive or all negative. Typically in a normal ECG they start as being negative in V_1 and V_2 and end up being positive in V_5 and V_6.

vi *The shape of the complex in V_1*: monophasic and biphasic complexes in V_1 favour ventricular tachycardia, whereas triphasic complexes ('M' or 'W' patterns) favour a supraventricular tachycardia, with the exception that a Rsr, triphasic pattern is more suggestive of a ventricular origin.

These factors may help in differentiating a ventricular tachycardia from a supraventricular tachycardia. However, if on the above evidence there is still diagnostic difficulty, always assume that the tachycardia is ventricular in origin.

In this man's case the fact that the tachycardia is ventricular in origin is supported by the following facts:

- He is 70 years old
- History of ischaemic heart disease
- Electrocardiographic features
  a Broad complexes of 0.14 s duration
  b Bizarre frontal plane axis, with a positive 'QRS' complex in AVR
  c Rsr pattern in V_1
  d Concordance across the chest leads
- Examination of the rhythm strip reveals no captured or fusion beats nor are there any obvious 'P' waves.

2 Immediate management

Always assume that a broad complex tachycardia is ventricular in origin.

- Place the patient on a couch, and attach him to a cardiac monitor
- Give oxygen
- Establish venous access
- Call senior help

- If the patient is haemodynamically stable, further consideration of the history, clinical examination and the electrocardiogram can aid in making a correct diagnosis

  If the patient is unstable, immediate treatment is necessary.

The treatment of sustained ventricular tachycardia

1 If no pulses present treat as ventricular fibrillation.
   a Call the resuscitation team
   ↓
   b Commence basic life support
   ↓
   c Charge the defibrillator and deliver:
   ↓
   200 joules
   ↓
   200 joules
   ↓
   360 joules
   ↓
   lignocaine 100 mg

and continue adhering to the Resuscitation Council (UK) guidelines for ventricular fibrillation until sinus rhythm is restored (see Case 32).

2 If a pulse is present: Call for senior help.

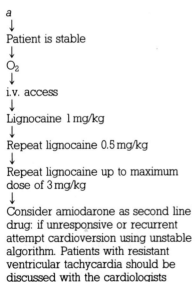

a	b
↓	↓
Patient is stable	Patient is unstable
↓	↓
O₂	O₂
↓	↓
i.v. access	i.v. access
↓	↓
Lignocaine 1 mg/kg	Sedation
↓	↓
Repeat lignocaine 0.5 mg/kg	Cardiovert 200 Joules
↓	↓
Repeat lignocaine up to maximum dose of 3 mg/kg	Cardiovert 200 Joules
↓	↓
Consider amiodarone as second line drug: if unresponsive or recurrent attempt cardioversion using unstable algorithm. Patients with resistant ventricular tachycardia should be discussed with the cardiologists	Cardiovert 360 Joules
	↓
	If unresponsive, use lignocaine in dose suggested in stable column. Second line drug amiodarone

Notes

a If the patient becomes unstable at any time, move to the unstable arm of the algorithm.

b Unstable would be implied by heart failure, hypotension (BP < 90 mmHg) or severe chest pain.

c Sedation (and therefore the presence of an anaesthetist) should be considered in all patients who are not unconscious.

d Once successfully terminated an infusion of the antiarrhythmic that aided in the resolution of the ventricular tachycardia should be started.

(Adapted from *Journal of the American Medical Association* (1986),**25**).

Practice points

A sustained episode of ventricular tachycardia does not necessarily lead to cardiovascular compromise.

In the absence of fusion or captured beats ventricular tachycardia is regular.

Being male, over 35 years old and with a past medical history of ischaemic heart disease or congestive cardiac failure is over 90% sensitive for a ventricular tachycardia.

If any doubt exists and the patient is unstable treat as ventricular tachycardia, if the patient is stable obtain a senior opinion before administering drugs.

References

Baerman, J. M., Morady, F., Dicarlo, L. A. *et al.* (1987) Differentiation of ventricular tachycardia from supraventricular tachycardia with aberration: value of the clinical history. *Annals of Emergency Medicine,* **16**, 40

Griffith, M. J. and Camm, J. (1989) Broad complex tachycardia. *Hospital Update,* 531–541

Levitt, M. A. (1988) Supraventricular tachycardia with aberrant conduction versus ventricular tachycardia. *American Journal of Emergency Medicine,* **6**, 273–277

Case 15

A 23-year-old estate agent injured his right knee while on a dry ski slope following a collision with another skier. He had been aware of acute pain in his right knee as he fell and heard a loud crack. He was unable to bear weight and was helped to his feet by friends. One hour later, when at home he treated his knee with elevation and a cold compress. The next morning the knee was swollen, stiff and painful, and his father drove him down to the local Accident and Emergency department.

In the past he had not had any knee problems though he had sprained his right ankle on a number of occasions playing football.

On examination:

- Unable to bear weight on his right knee
- Right knee was swollen
- Obvious effusion with a patella tap
- Active range of movement was very limited and he preferred to keep his knee slightly flexed over a pillow
- There was medial joint line tenderness with some minimal bruising
- Pain limited further examination including assessing the stability of the knee
- Radiographic examination confirmed the presence of an effusion but no fracture line was visible

Questions

1 What further points in the history is it important to elicit?
2 What is your management?

Answers

1 Further history

Further history should include details of (a) the mechanism of injury, and (b) an indication of how quickly the knee became swollen.

a The mechanism of injury is very important. From the presumed stresses applied to the knee at the time of injury an indication of the structures likely to be damaged can be obtained. In this man an idea of the direction of the collision and how he fell in relation to his skis would give some idea of the direction of the force applied to the knee during the injury. Table 2 indicates the structures likely to be damaged in the knee when the direction of force is known. (In children fractures through the epiphysis, may simulate ligamentous injuries, and in the elderly, ligamentous injuries are often associated with fractures of osteoporotic bone.)

b How quickly did the knee become swollen? In the acutely injured knee swelling that occurs within the first 6 h is due to blood. An acute haemarthrosis always indicates the possibility of serious intra-articular damage. The bleeding is due to damage to the synovium, ligaments or bone, or any combination of these three. Conversely, a joint that becomes swollen 12 h or more after the injury will be an inflammatory reaction of the synovium to a non-specific insult, and will consequently be straw-coloured rather than blood stained. It is difficult to be sure on

Table 2 Structures damaged in the knee when direction of force is known.
(Forces described as being applied to the tibia)

Valgus force (Car bumper injury is a typical mechanism)	Medial collateral ligament Medial meniscus Anterior cruciate ligament Posterior cruciate ligament
Varus force (Less common than valgus injury as other leg tends to protect from this type of injury)	Lateral collateral ligament Lateral meniscus Posterior cruciate Anterior cruciate
Hyperextension (A blow to the front of the knee)	Anterior cruciate Posterior cruciate
Posterior displacement in flexion (knee hitting dashboard)	Posterior cruciate Anterior cruciate
Internal rotation (External rotation of the trunk, when the foot is fixed as in sports)	Anterior cruciate Posterior cruciate Lateral collateral ligament
External rotation (Sports and skiing)	Medial collateral ligament Lateral collateral ligament Meniscus

clinical grounds what the nature of an effusion which takes an intermediate amount of time to develop (6–12 h). Aspiration of the joint resolves this difficulty.

This man was able to describe that he was hit from behind and he was knocked forwards. However, his right ski was trapped in the other person's skis. This arrested his forward progress, he twisted around (external rotation of the tibia on the femur) and he fell to the ground. The effusion was noticed when he awoke 10 h after the accident, but with hindsight he was aware that the knee was slightly swollen before he went to bed.

2 Management

Management consists of (see Figure 5):

a *Aspiration of the joint*
   Pain and discomfort limit the full assessment of this man's knee. The injury appears significant in that he has not been able to bear weight on his knee since the accident, and the likelihood is that he has a haemarthrosis. The knee needs to be aspirated as this will not only confirm the presence of blood, but may also reduce the discomfort and allow a more formal assessment of the intra-articular structures.

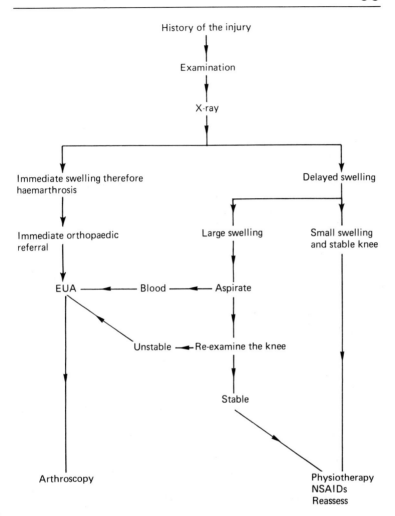

Figure 5 Algorithm for the management of the acutely swollen knee

When aspirating the knee joint, as with any joint, scrupulous aseptic technique is necessary.

110 ml of frank blood was aspirated, with considerable symptomatic relief for the patient.

b *Re-assess the stability of the knee*

Instability of the knee should now be assessed by testing the integrity of all the intra-articular ligaments.

i *Valgus and varus stability*: assessment of the collateral ligaments.

In full extension, and then in 20° of flexion, varus and valgus forces should be applied to the knee. Instability demonstrated in full extension raises the possibility of not only collateral ligament injury, but also cruciate injury, as all ligaments are taut in full extension. At 20° of flexion the collaterals only are stressed as the cruciates, ability to resist valgus and varus forces are lost as the knee flexes.

ii *Anterior drawer test*: assessment of the stability of the anterior cruciate ligament.

This is performed with the knee in 90° of flexion. The examiner sits upon the foot, immobilizing it, and the tibia is passively drawn forward with the hamstring muscles relaxed; an abnormal degree of movement is noted in the affected knee.

Other clinical test for anterior cruciate instability are said to be useful, such as the pivot shift test, but experience is needed to perform them and interpret the results.

iii *Posterior sag test*: assessment of the posterior cruciate ligament.

With the knees in 90° of flexion as for the anterior drawer test, the contour of each knee is observed. Damage, to the posterior cruciate ligament allows the tibia to sag back on the femur, altering the profile of the knee when compared with normal.

iv *McMurray's test*: assessment of the menisci.

This test assesses the integrity of the menisci; a positive test is useful, but a negative result does not exclude injury. It is performed with the finger tips of one hand placed on the joint line overlying the menisci. The other hand grasps the heel and rotates the tibia on the femur throughout the permitted range of flexion. An audible click, pronounced discomfort or grating sensation would all suggest meniscal injury.

In this man a significant give and pain was produced when a valgus stress was applied to his knee in 20° of flexion raising the possibility of medial collateral ligament damage.

This patient has presented with an acute haemarthrosis and instability of the medial collateral ligament. He needs to be referred immediately to the orthopaedics team on duty.

Arthroscopy (and examination under anaesthetic (EUA) are particularly useful in the management of the acutely injured knee. This is because the clinical examination of the acutely injured knee is notoriously inaccurate.

Arthroscopy performed in the presence of a haemarthrosis reveals a clinically significant injury in over 90% of patients. By far the commonest injury associated with an haemarthrosis is rupture of anterior cruciate ligament which is found in 70% of cases, either in isolation or in association with meniscal injuries, or capsular tears. Finding multiple injuries is common, and hence arthroscopy is necessary for accurate evaluation of every haemarthrosis.

Be aware of the patient with a very bruised knee and no obvious haemarthrosis. Damage to the joint capsule may have allowed the effusion to track into the tissues around the knee.

Outcome

This man was admitted and underwent arthroscopy. He was found to have a tear in the medial collateral ligament, a torn anterior cruciate, and small tear in the medial meniscus – the so-called O'Donohue's triad. These lesions were repaired at open operation.

Practice points

1 As with all musculoskeletal injuries, an appreciation of the exact mechanism of injury is important in making a correct diagnosis.
2 There is a clinically significant injury in over 90% of all haemarthroses. All haemarthroses therefore should be referred for orthopaedic assessment.
3 Aspiration of large effusions provides symptomatic relief and can aid the diagnosis by either confirming the presence of blood, or by allowing a more thorough examination of the knee.

Case 16

A 75-year-old woman brought to Accident and Emergency by ambulance was comatose. Her husband was able to relate the following history. She had been hypertensive for many years for which she received medication, and 3 years prior to presentation she had developed a left-sided weakness which had resolved completely over 3 months. That evening she had suddenly sat down while ironing and complained of a headache, vertigo and nausea and then collapsed to the ground and went limp. She did not fit, and as she remained unresponsive the husband called the ambulance. Other than tablets for mild diabetes there was no significant history.

On examination:

- Airway clear
- Periodic respiration (Cheynes Stokes) at 16/min
- Pyrexial 37.8°C
- Pulse 100/min, blood pressure 190/110 mmHg
- Chest – right basal crepitations
- Abdomen soft, bowel sounds present

- No evidence of trauma to head, or elsewhere
- No eye opening to pain
- No verbal response to pain
- Withdrew all four limbs to pain
- Pupils pinpoint and unreactive to light
- Doll's head eye movements absent
- Oculovestibular reflex absent
- Gag reflex absent
- Corneal reflexes absent
- No neck stiffness
- Flaccid limbs, reflexes; diminished on the left (asymmetrical)
- Extensor plantar responses

Questions

1 What is the emergency management?
2 What is her Glasgow coma score?
3 Where is the lesion?
4 What are the possible diagnoses?

Answers

1 See Appendix

2 Glasgow coma score

This woman's coma score is 6.

3 Site of lesion

The brainstem or posterior fossa.

4 Diagnosis

This hypertensive woman suddenly became comatose, after a brief prodrome of headache, vertigo and nausea. The sudden mode of onset is very suggestive of a vascular incident. The loss of brainstem reflexes from the outset of the coma suggest a subtentorial lesion. The periodic respiratory pattern and the pin-point pupils suggest damage to the pontine region of the brainstem.

In practice vascular lesions are the commonest cause, with either haemorrhage into, or infarction of, the brainstem, or compression of the brainstem by a cerebellar haematoma.

If there was evidence of a head injury then these brainstem signs would suggest a posterior fossa subdural or extradural haematoma.

Although this history given is typical for a pontine haemorrhage, vascular lesions can affect any part of the brainstem. Clinical features will vary depending on the site involved, but all will have a combination of the following – pupillary changes, abnormal respiratory pattern, abnormal eye movements and asymmetrical long tract signs. Brainstem vascular events most commonly occur in hypertensive elderly patients. There may have been a history of, or previous transient ischaemia of the brainstem giving rise to symptoms such as vertigo, diplopia, dysarthria, dysphagia and drop attacks.

There is little active treatment that can be offered to patients with brainstem strokes. However, a cerebellar haematoma which by external compression of the brainstem can mimic the signs may respond to surgical drainage if the condition is recognized early.

Cerebellar haematomas develop in patients with hypertension, a-v-malformations. The prodromal symptoms are exactly like those of impending brainstem vascular occlusion. However, deterioration is slower, it usually takes several hours for the brainstem signs to develop. Once the patient is comatose the outcome of surgical evacuation is poor.

Outcome

The clinical diagnosis was of a brainstem vascular accident. This patient became progressively more comatose and then apnoeic. She was not resuscitated.

Reference

Plum, F. and Posner, J. B. (1980) *Diagnosis of Stupor and Coma.* 3rd edn. F. A. Davis Co., Philadelphia, 9

Case 17

A mother brought her 4-year-old daughter to the Accident and Emergency department because she would not bear weight on her left leg. She had been limping the day before, and complained of pain in her knee. Today she had refused to use the leg at all. Three days previously she had developed a cough and a fever and had not been well enough to attend playschool. She had become listless, irritable, anorectic and vomited twice. Her mother had administered Calpol regularly. There had been no history of trauma to the leg, and no significant past medical history.

On examination:

- Child looked unwell
- Pyrexial 38.2°C
- Runny nose, red throat, pink ear drums
- Enlarged cervical lymph nodes
- Chest clear
- Abdomen soft
- There was marked muscle spasm preventing movement of the left hip, a reduced range of movements, in particular flexion, abduction and internal rotation, when compared with the right hip
- Movement of the knees and ankles were normal and non-tender
- There was no evidence of trauma
- The rest of the examination was normal

Questions

1 What is the significance of the knee pain?
2 What is the diagnosis?
3 What is your management?

Answers

1 Lesions of the hip joint can give rise to pain felt exclusively in the anterior thigh and knee. This is referred pain from the joint via the second and third lumbar segments. Not appreciating this fact may trap the unwary.

In some infants it may be impossible to localize the pain and it may be necessary to have radiographs of the whole limb.

2 The most likely diagnosis is transient synovitis of the hip (irritable hip). This condition, which may be recurrent, can affect children from 2 to 12 years old. The aetiology is not well understood but often presents during or after a mild coryzal illness with a limp and a degree of loss of movement at the joint which may vary from acute spasm with all movements being limited to mild restriction of movement.

The main differential diagnosis is septic arthritis. This condition, although much less common, is much more serious and needs intensive treatment. It should be considered in children with very marked hip spasm, who are pyrexial and unwell.

Perthes' disease of the hip is a possibility. Although it may present in this fashion, the diagnosis would be made retrospectively as often there are no diagnostic features at initial presentation. It is uncommon before the age of four and has a preponderance for males.

3 Management should include:

i Radiographs of both hip joints – may demonstrate a joint effusion.
ii Full blood count – a leucocytosis would be expected in septic arthritis.
iii ESR – elevated in septic arthritis.
iv Blood cultures.
v Ultrasound examination – ultrasound is being used more frequently to look for effusions in these children.
vi The child needs referral to the orthopaedic team for admission and exclusion of septic arthritis.

Children with mild restriction of movement, who can walk and are constitutionally well and apyrexial, can be discharged and advised to rest the affected limb until the pain settles. Early review of these children is necessary, 24–48 h by the orthopaedic team.

Outcome

This child was taken to theatre for aspiration of the hip joint under general anaesthesia. The aspirate was sterile. The child made a dramatic recovery over the next 24 h and was allowed home.

Reference

Cyriax, J. (1983) *Textbook of Orthopaedic Medicine.* Vol 1. 8th edn. Diagnosis of soft tissue lesions. Baillière Tindall, London

Case 18

A 28-year-old male was found in the street by a passerby in a drowsy but rousable state. An ambulance brought him to the department by which time he was fully orientated and awake. He gave a history of being completely well that morning, but on the way to a local sandwich bar for lunch he suddenly experienced a great whooshing noise in his head which lasted for 30 s. There was no associated pain. Then he was aware of someone apparently asking him directions, but on looking around no one was there. The last thing he remembers was a strange tingling sensation which started in his abdomen and rose through his chest to his head and neck. The next recollection he had was being on the ground and a passerby asking him whether he was alright. He was aware that he had bitten his tongue during the episode. Now he felt much better but rather tired.

He recalled an episode 3 weeks previously of hearing voices and total body tingling which was very short lived lasting only 10 s or so, he had put this down to the pressure of work.

In the past there was no history of psychiatric disease, chronic ear problems, or drugs. There was no family history of epilepsy and he had never had a fit before.

On examination:

- Well, apyrexial
- Orientated time, place and person
- Glasgow coma score 15
- His behaviour and speech content were appropriate
- He was anxious but had good insight
- Thought content was normal
- He appeared intelligent and although concentration was mildly impaired his memory was good
- There was no external evidence of head injury
- Both ear drums were normal
- There were no focal neurological signs or evidence of meningism
- BM stick estimation 4–7 mmol/l
- The remainder of the examination was normal

Questions

1 What is the diagnosis and management?
2 What further advice should be given to the patient?

Answers

1 Diagnosis and management

The most likely diagnosis is focal epilepsy starting in the temporal lobe and progressing to a generalized convulsion. The evidence of tongue biting and postictal drowsiness are very suggestive that the loss of consciousness was due to a convulsion. The temporal lobe is the commonest site for a focal epileptiform discharge (partial seizure) and some may progress to a generalized seizure.

Common symptoms in temporal lobe epilepsy are vague abdominal discomfort rising through the chest to the head, sensations of fear, déjâ vu and jamais vu, complex chewing and sucking actions and olfactory and visual hallucinations. Auditory hallucinations are less common but well recognized.

Other conditions which may present in a similar way are herpes simplex encephalitis, amphetamine abuse and psychiatric disorders.

Herpes simplex encephalitis may be a rapidly fatal condition which can present with temporal lobe symptoms, fits, confusion and signs of meningeal irritation. Because of the progressive nature of the disease patients are unwell from the outset and deteriorate. The fact that this patient has completely recovered from the fit, is apyrexial without any meningeal signs, and had a similar episode 3 weeks previously excludes the diagnosis.

There is no suspicion that this man has a formal thought disorder on clinical examination and this would be an unusual presentation for depression or schizophrenia.

As the fit was focal initially a CT scan of the brain is necessary to exclude a space-occupying lesion. Referral to the duty medical team.

Outcome

The duty neurological registrar confirmed that a focal temporal seizure progressing to a generalized convulsion was the most likely diagnosis.

A CT scan was organized as an outpatient and the patient discharged on an increasing dose of carbamazepine.

2 Further advice

The patient should be advised that he should no longer drive; he should inform the DVLA that he has had a fit. This could be devastating for the patient if he drives regularly for work purposes, but failure to inform the patient of his legal duty could result in lethal consequences (for which you may be judged liable). Advice should also be given about activities such as roofing, working on scaffolding etc., swimming, rock climbing, bicycle riding etc.

Further notes

The management of a patient with a first fit

People who have a convulsion in public are often brought to Accident and Emergency departments.

Many patients will feel normal within 2 or 3 h. Most patients may be safely discharged provided:

1 Full recovery has occurred, and the patient is alert and orientated when examined.
2 They are asymptomatic, and clinical examination is normal, in particular, they are apyrexial, without evidence of meningeal irritation, and there are no focal signs.
3 They are not hypoglycaemic.
4 They have not sustained a significant head injury.
5 They will be in the presence of a responsible adult.

Patients should be discharged home with a letter for their general practitioner, and an urgent neurology outpatient appointment. If possible an EEG should be arranged so that the results can be reviewed when the patient is seen.

Advice about driving and sporting activities should be re-emphasized.

Reference

Springings, D. and Chambers, J. (1990) *Acute Medicine*. Blackwell Scientific Publications, Oxford

Case 19

A 24-year-old male presented with a 36-h history of lower back pain. He worked as an operating department assistant (ODA) and had suddenly developed the pain 2 days previously when lifting a patient off the operating table onto a trolley. The pain radiated into his buttocks and down both legs. He was unable to continue working and was sent home with the advice to rest in bed. Four months previously he had had a similar episode of lower back pain, without the leg symptoms. This initial episode was again precipitated by lifting. He had spent a week in bed and it had spontaneously resolved.

During this episode, the pain was becoming progressively worse, and was exacerbated by movement and coughing. He indicated that the pain radiated down the posterior lateral aspects of both thighs, around the lateral side of the calves and into the dorsum of both feet. As he lived alone he was finding it increasingly difficult to cope at home. He had never suffered with back pain before starting as an ODA, and was otherwise well.

On examination:

- Obese. In pain
- Respiratory rate 18/min; blood pressure 130/90 mmHg; pulse 88/min
- Chest clear
- Abdomen soft
- Straight leg raising was limited, right to 50°, left to 30°
- Straight leg raising was more limited if the test was repeated with the foot dorsiflexed
- Weakness of extension of left big toe
- Hypoaesthesia in the first interspace on the left
- There were no other neurological signs in the legs

He found it very difficult to get off the trolley and stood stooped supporting himself against the wall. Back movements, flexion, extension and lateral flexion were severely limited. He was unable to walk on his heels, but was able to walk around on his tip toes. He was unable to sit down, as this exacerbated the pain in his legs.

Questions

1 What is the probable diagnosis?
2 What further history and examination is necessary?
3 Compression of which nerve root would give rise to the signs in the left leg?
4 What is your management?

Answers

1 The clinical diagnosis is central prolapse of an intervertebral disc giving rise to bilateral symptoms of nerve root compression.

2 A central disc protrusion gives rise to pressure on the cauda equina and thereby may give rise to compression of multiple nerve roots, both lumbar and sacral. This may result in loss of sphincter control. It is always important therefore to enquire about sphincter disturbance in any patient with lower back pain. Clinical examination should always include an assessment of perianal sensation, anal sphincter tone and eliciting the anal reflex. Acute lesions affecting the cauda equina, if not recognized and treated promptly, may result in a permanent impairment of sphincter control.

3 Nerve root compression in the back gives rise to symptoms in the affected dermatome. Pain, paraesthesia and loss of function may be present. This man has symptoms of L5 nerve compression in both legs, though motor signs are limited to the left leg. (See Table 3 for signs of nerve root compression.)

4 Symptoms of bladder disturbance should be sought, further examination for saddle anaesthesia, and assessment of the anal reflex and tone should be performed. The man should be nursed flat.

- Analgesia given (diclofenac sodium 75 mg i.m.)
- Lumbar spine radiographs requested
- Refer to the orthopaedic team

Outcome

There was no history of sphincter disturbance, and there were no further clinical signs on examination. A CT myelogram demonstrated a central disc prolapse at L4,5. This was removed at operation, and the man made an uneventful recovery.

Further notes

Assessment of back pain in the Accident and Emergency department

Back pain is very common. It is estimated that 80% of the adult population will experience back pain at some time during their lives, and it is the second most common ailment cited keeping people off work. As a consequence it is a condition commonly seen in the Accident and Emergency departments. A simple structured approach is necessary to ensure adequate evaluation of all patients.

History

Below are some common causes of back pain, with a typical presenting history.

1 *Acute back strain.* An overweight man plays a golf match for charity though he rarely takes any exercise. He presents the next day with low back pain, which was exacerbated if he simulated his golf swing.

2 *Chronic back strain* and
3 *Degenerative disc disease.* Both these conditions give rise to chronic intermittent pain. The symptoms are typically provoked by activities such as injudicious lifting. The discomfort may be experienced in the buttocks or back of the thighs, but not below the knee.

4 *Prolapsed intervertebral disc.* Acute episodes of disc prolapse with radicular symptoms give rise to quite typical symptoms. A patient develops acute back pain suddenly while doing something active, followed by pain or paraesthesia experienced in the thigh, leg and foot. The initiating insult can be quite trivial, and there is usually a history of previous intermittent self-limiting back pain. Radicular symptoms are suggested by a history of pain experienced below the knee. Pain limited to the buttocks or thighs is usually thought of as being referred in nature.

5 *Cauda equina syndrome.* The onset of back pain, with radicular symptoms in both legs, associated perineal pain, or sphincter disturbance should always make you suspicious of a central disc prolapse.

6 *Crush fracture of lumbar vertebra.* An elderly woman develops sudden back pain, usually in the lumbar spine after a relatively minor episode of trauma. The pain is constant, exacerbated by movement and often gives rise to referred pain.

7 *Atypical pain.* Remember that in particular renal, pancreatic and vascular conditions may present with back pain. Always enquire about urinary symptoms, and obtain a vascular history (claudication, hypertension). Renal calculi and aneurysms may give rise to pain which

may be thought to be musculoskeletal in origin. Remember, a history of unremitting back pain, which is worse at night is suggestive of bone pain (infection, malignancy).

The examination

Ideally all patients should be examined both lying and standing. Pain may limit the examination and it is often helpful to wait until the analgesia you prescribed has had time to work (diclofenac sodium 75 mg i.m./p.r. is useful). The vast majority of patients with back pain will be cared for as outpatients, and it is imperative that they are examined, standing, when their mobility and gait can be assessed.

The range of back movements, muscular spasm and local tenderness are most readily appreciated by standing behind the patient. Their ability to walk on tip toes, and then on their heels, assesses gross motor power in L4,5 and S1,2. Their ability to climb onto the couch and lie down also gives a useful clinical guide to how severe their symptoms are and how well they will be able to manage at home.

In the supine position, straight leg raising is readily performed. If straight leg raising is limited by pain which radiates below the knee then this is indicative of nerve root compression. However, more often than not it is limited by tightness and discomfort in the hamstring muscles which is normal and varies with the degree of suppleness of the patient. If radicular pain is exacerbated by straight leg raising, then the test should be repeated, this time with the foot dorsiflexed. This should further limit the degree of straight leg raising as it stretches the nerve. Reproducing the radicular pain in the affected leg by attempting straight leg raising in the unaffected leg is a convincing sign of a true radiculopathy.

Power and tone should then be assessed in all muscle groups, the reflexes should be elicited and sensation, including perianal, should be documented. Although more than one nerve root may be compressed at any one time, symptoms usually predominate in a single root giving rise to a typical distribution of symptoms and signs.

Most commonly, disc lesions occur at L4,5 and L5,S1 and affect the roots L5 and S1 respectively. Less commonly, L3,4 disc gives rise to L4 radicular symptoms, however disc lesions above L4 are uncommon and alternative pathologies should be suspected.

For the signs see Table 3.

The abdomen should be palpated for masses, and in particular an aortic aneurysm which may present with back pain in the elderly. Tenderness in the renal angles should be sought.

With the patient then in the prone position, the femoral nerve stretch test should be performed. With the knee flexed, the hip should be extended, if this elicits pain then a L4 radiculopathy should be suspected.

It is also possible directly to palpate the sacroiliac joints in this position.

The examination is not complete without urinanalysis.

Table 3 Signs of nerve root compression

	L4	L5	S1	Cauda equina
Pain	Posterior lateral thigh, and anterior medial leg down to medial malleolus	Back of thigh. Lateral leg and dorsum of the foot	Posterior thigh and leg to heel and lateral foot	Bilateral leg pain and/or perineal pain
Sensory loss	Medial leg	Dorsum of the foot and 1st interspace	Lateral sole of foot	Perineal and/or bilateral leg
Weakness	Quadriceps. Extension of the knee and inversion of the foot	Dorsiflexion of great toe/ and foot. Difficulty walking on heel	Planter flexion and eversion of foot. Difficulty walking on toes	Variable, includes sphincter disturbance
Reflex arc	Knee jerk diminished	Nil	Ankle jerk	Ankle jerk

Cautionary tale
A woman of 50 presented with atypical back pain of 3-month's duration, with features of chronic back strain. There were no renal symptoms. Urinanalysis revealed blood + + +. A plain X-ray of the abdomen, including the kidneys, ureters and bladder demonstrated a huge staghorn calculus in her left kidney. This was removed by open operation with relief of her symptoms.

X-ray examination

Radiographs of the lumbar spine are time consuming and often contribute very little useful information to the management of many patients, although the following patients should have radiographs taken:

- History suggestive of bone pain
- History of significant trauma
- History of acute on chronic pain
- Neurological signs
- The elderly (crush fractures, malignancy)

Management

The majority of patients should be managed as outpatients. Strict bed rest and non-steroidal anti-inflammatory drugs (NSAIDs) being the mainstay of treatment.
    The following patients should be referred for admission:

1 All patients with recent onset of neurological signs.
2 Severe pain severely limiting mobility in a patient who lives alone.
3 History of sphincter disturbance, even in the absence of clinical signs.
4 Crush fractures in the elderly – if management as an outpatient not feasible because of pain, or lack of support, or if the fracture is potentially unstable (i.e. more than 50% reduction in the size of the vertebra).

Reference

Frymoyer, J. (1988) Back pain and sciatica. *New England Journal of Medicine,* **318,** 291–298

Case 20

A 15-year-old girl was running across an ornamental garden when she slipped and fell headlong into a flower bed. There was a small 1 foot (30 cm) high wall around the flower bed on which she fell injuring her lower chest and upper abdomen. She cried out in pain, and had appeared to have 'winded' herself. As she failed to get better after 10 min, and looked very pale, her friends called for an ambulance. Twenty minutes after the fall she was on the way to hospital. No other history was available.

On examination:

- Conscious, talking but confused
- Pale
- Respiratory rate was 28/min
- There were no obvious external signs of injury to chest or abdomen
- Both sides of the chest moved normal, and air entry was equal bilaterally
- The trachea was central
- Her peripheries were pale, and cold, and her radial pulse was not palpable
- Heart rate 140/min
- Her femoral pulse was palpable, but her blood pressure was unrecordable
- The abdomen was soft, not distended and bowel sounds were present
- External compression of the pelvis elicited no tenderness, crepitus or movement
- Examination of the external genitalia revealed an intact hymen
- There was no obvious external injury elsewhere, to the limbs, head or to the back

Questions

1 What is the working diagnosis?
2 What is your immediate management?

Answers

1 Diagnosis

The working diagnosis is profound hypovolaemic shock. The hypovolaemic shock is secondary to intra-abdominal bleeding. In the traumatized patient concealed haemorrhage producing shock may occur in the chest, abdomen or pelvis. This injury was a relatively low energy impact of the lower thoracic cage and upper abdomen against a solid structure. It would be highly unlikely for such an injury to cause a major disruption of the pelvis and clinically from the initial assessment this is excluded. Clinical examination failed to reveal any obvious external injury, or any signs in the chest compatible with a large haemothorax or tension pneumothorax. The upper abdominal organs, the liver and spleen, lie beneath the costal margin, the site of injury, and both are liable to be the source of brisk haemorrhage when injured. In adults the overlying lower ribs are often broken by the force which causes the visceral damage, in children and young adults however the chest wall is much more compliant and can absorb a greater amount of energy before rib fracture occurs.

Do not be fooled by the lack of abdominal signs or by the presence of bowel sounds in the presence of intra-abdominal injury. Up to 20% of patients with significant abdominal injury have no abnormal abdominal signs when first seen in Accident and Emergency. Likewise, normal bowel sounds may persist after injury and these should never be used to exclude intra-abdominal injury.

A ruptured ectopic pregnancy should always be considered as a possibility in shocked females of reproductive age. However, the intact hymen excludes this as a possible diagnosis.

The nature and site of the injury giving rise to intra-abdominal haemorrhage is less important than realizing that the patient is bleeding and that the patient's condition cannot be explained by injury elsewhere.

Numerically the spleen is more likely to be the cause of haemorrhage, however the Royal College of Surgeons Report (1989) found that of patients who died as a result of unsuspected abdominal haemorrhage the liver was a commoner site of the bleeding than the spleen.

2 Immediate management

This girl has many of the typical features of severe hypovolaemic shock. The trauma team (senior Accident and Emergency staff, duty surgeon and the anaesthetist) should be called directly, and the operating theatre and blood transfusion informed.

Immediate management consists of:

Airway: patients that are able to talk do not have an obstructed airway, but as with all traumatized patients 60% oxygen via Venturi mask is necessary.

Cervical spine: this should be immobilized in a rigid collar.

Breathing: the chest should be examined to exclude it as the site of massive haemorrhage, and other conditions which may give rise to profound shock, i.e. tension pneumothorax.

Circulation: the pallor, confusion, cold peripheries and delayed capillary return (normal 2 s) all suggest hypoperfusion. The pulse rate of 140/min and the undetectable blood pressure suggest over 40% of circulating blood volume may have been lost. Pulse pressure falls with progressive hypovolaemia and blood pressures may be difficult to measure, using a cuff. A useful clinical guide for approximate blood pressure estimations are:

the presence of a radial pulse > 80 mmHg
the presence of a femoral pulse > 70 mmHg
the presence of a carotid pulse > 60 mmHg.

The priority here is to restore the circulating blood volume with blood (or colloid and crystalloid until blood is available). Two large bore (at least

14 gauge) cannulas should be sited, one in either antecubital fossa and a 2 l bolus of fluid given. Blood should be taken when siting the drip for urgent crossmatch of at least 6 units of blood, and due to the severity of hypovolaemia 4 units of uncrossmatched blood should be requested for initial management.

The bladder should be catheterized, and urine output measured. A nasogastric tube should be inserted, and the patient attached to a cardiac monitor.

Immediate preparations should be made to take the girl to theatre. Active resuscitation should continue on the way. A pneumatic antishock garment, if available could be applied as theatre is being prepared. Further management depends upon the response to the fluid bolus. A 2 l fluid challenge using two 14 gauge cannulas can be completed in 6 min. If there is little or no response to the fluid challenge, it suggests that bleeding is occurring at least as quickly as the fluid is being given, and immediate operative intervention is necessary.

If there is a dramatic response to fluid administration, with restoration of a good blood pressure and a decrease in the pulse rate with an improvement in the patient's general condition you have bought yourself a few extra minutes to allow full resuscitation with blood, before operation.

Peritoneal lavage (see p. 121) is contraindicated in this girl, as there is an *absolute indication for urgent laparotomy.*

Outcome

In this girl there was no response to fluid administration. Her abdomen although still soft was now very distended. She was taken to theatre, where it was found that the liver was the source of the bleeding. There were multiple lacerations of the liver parenchyma, and disruption of the hepatic veins. Despite extensive surgery and resuscitation the child died on the operating table.

Further notes

Fluid administration

The rate of flow is dependent upon the size and length of the cannula and not the vein (short wide cannulas are best). The longer the cannula the slower the rate of flow, which is why peripheral cannulas are preferable to long central lines for shock therapy. However, central venous measurement is necessary when large quantities of fluid are needed in resuscitation, especially in the elderly, and patients with pre-existing cardiac disease.

The response to the fluid bolus can be variable depending upon the rate of bleeding. One of three responses is usual.

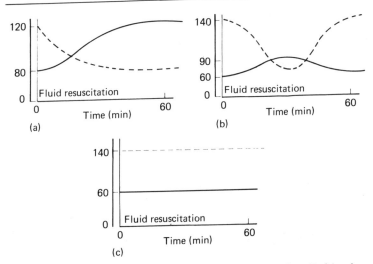

Figure 6 Pulse and blood pressure response to fluids. — Systolic blood pressure; – – – heart rate. (Courtesy of BMJ Publications)

1 There is a good response which is maintained. That is the patient is no longer bleeding, and initial losses have been corrected (Figure 6a).
2 There is a transient response which is not maintained. Initial losses are partially corrected, but the patient continues to bleed. The patient needs surgical intervention (Figure 6b).
3 There is no appreciable response at all, suggesting that the patient continues to bleed, at least as quickly as fluid is given. The patient needs immediate surgical intervention. (Ensure that causes of profound shock other than hypovolaemia have been excluded, Figure 6c.)

When venous access is a problem

The antecubital fossa is the best place to site a cannula. The course and position of the big veins here are known to all doctors, but any site in the arm will do so long as large cannulas are used. Failing this, the long saphenous vein at the ankle is a useful site. Otherwise either a cut down, or central line/femoral line insertion (short, wide cannula) will be necessary. Cut downs are most easily performed either in the antecubital fossa, or on to the long saphenous vein at the ankle.

The site of these veins *are*:

1 Long saphenous: approximately 2 cm anterior and superior to the medial malleolus.
2 Medial basilic vein: 2.5 cm lateral to the medial epicondyle of the humerus at the flexion crease of the elbow.

Recognizing hypovolaemic shock

The initial signs of hypovolaemic shock are subtle. Many victims of major trauma are young, without pre-existing cardiopulmonary disease, and are quite capable of compensating for loss of up to 30% of their circulating blood volume without dropping their blood pressure. Early signs of hypovolaemia are:

- *Tachypnoea* usually not noted, as we are poor at monitoring the respiratory rate.
- *Tachycardia* often attributed to pain and anxiety.
- *Anxiety and sweating* often manifest as fright, or hostility.
- *Decreased pulse pressure* there is a rise in the diastolic pressure.

Over 30% of blood volume lost produces a drop in systolic blood pressure, a significant tachycardia of greater than 120/min, and confusion, in short the changes in the physiological parameters which many of us need to diagnose active bleeding. More than 40% of blood volume lost produces a marked tachycardia (>140/min), and very low, or difficult to measure blood pressure (<80 mmHg) and marked depression of the mental state.

Over 50% results in loss of consciousness, pulse and blood pressure. Prompt resuscitation and early surgical intervention are the mainstays of treatment.

Always be vigilant when faced with the acutely injured patient, and do not ignore the subtle signs of active bleeding.

Cautionary tales

A man of 20 was hit by a bus while crossing the road. On arrival at hospital he was conscious, and complained of pain in this left thigh. Clinical and radiological examination revealed a fracture of the left femur as being the only apparent injury. His blood pressure was 125/70 mmHg and pulse was 118/min. He was placed in traction and sent to the orthopaedic ward. Within 5 minutes of being on the ward he suddenly collapsed with a pulse rate of 140/min and an unrecordable blood pressure, quickly arrested, and despite intensive resuscitation died. Post mortem revealed a ruptured spleen.

It was only the tachycardia which indicated active bleeding during the initial assessment, the abdominal examination being normal.

A young man, was hit by a vehicle, and was found confused and abusive by the side of the road by the ambulance staff. He became progresively more aggressive on arriving in the Accident and Emergency department, not allowing anyone near him. He then suddenly collapsed. He was cold, clammy, sweaty with a tachycardia and an unrecordable blood pressure. He failed to respond to initial fluid therapy and despite early operation died from a shattered liver.

References

Driscoll, P., Skinner, D. and Earlham, R. (eds) (1991) *ABC of Major Trauma*. BMJ Publications, London

Royal College of Surgeons (1988) *British Medical Journal*, **296**, 1305. Retrospective study of 1000 deaths from injury in England and Wales

Case 21

A woman of 32 years woke with acute pain in the shoulder, and was aware that she had been incontinent of urine. There was no previous history of epilepsy or of shoulder or neck problems.

On examination:

- Well. The shoulder looked normal
- All movements at the shoulder were painful and severely limited, especially external rotation.

Question

What is the diagnosis?

Answer

The diagnosis is a posterior dislocation of the right shoulder. Posterior dislocation is a well recognized complication of a tonic/clonic convulsion. The shoulder dislocates during the tonic phase as the arms are forcibly internally rotated. The incontinence is the clue to the probable fit. As with an anterior dislocation of the shoulder, posterior dislocation is acutely painful and leads to a severe reduction of all movements of the shoulder, in particular external rotation.

The clinical signs of posterior dislocation are subtle but constant. The shoulder contour is altered, a fact more readily appreciated from above, as the posteriorly dislocated humeral head produces a visible and palpable posterior prominence. The AP radiograph may appear normal, though the 'light-bulb' appearance of the internally rotated humeral head is characteristic. To exclude the diagnosis a second film is imperative, and an axillary view should be requested. It is often difficult to obtain a proper axillary view and a modified view will usually suffice. Entonox is helpful during positioning of the shoulder for this view.

Reduction is usually simple to achieve by applying traction to the abducted (90°) arm and then externally rotating it. If the reduction is stable, the shoulder should be rested in a sling and the patient reviewed in the orthoapedic clinic.

If however the shoulder will not stay reduced, advice from the orthopaedic team is necessary.

For further management of a first fit see p. 61.

Reference

Vickers, R. (1991) *Journal of the Medical Defence Union*, 1, 9

Case 22

A man brought his 28-year-old wife to the Accident and Emergency department as he was concerned about her behaviour. They had moved to the area 3 weeks ago because he had changed his job. During the first week in their new home he had noticed that his wife was increasingly anxious and suspicious of the neighbours. She found it difficult to sleep and was constantly moving the furniture around the bedroom during the early hours of the morning. When questioned about this she told her husband that the neighbours had moved them when they were asleep. During the second week she became increasingly anxious about leaving the flat to go shopping as she knew the neighbours would be in to 'interfere' with the furniture. Her sleep became increasingly disturbed, she had stopped eating, and complained that the neighbours were now calling her names.

The man explained that he had found the neighbours both helpful and pleasant. He was sure that they were neither entering their flat nor talking about his wife.

He had been prompted to seek help at this time because on returning from work he had discovered his wife standing on a chair by the open window. She told him that the 'voices' were telling her to jump out of the window as she was worthless.

There was no history of previous mental or physical illness, and she did not take any regular medication. She denied drinking heavily or taking drugs.

Her mother had died 4 months previously which had upset her profoundly, and she had felt unable to work since.

On examination:

- Well dressed
- Kept playing with jewellery, was startled by every extraneous noise and kept looking towards the door
- Unable to sit still, constantly pacing around the room
- Eye contact good

Below are the most illuminating answers that she gave during the mental state examination.

'I can't stay in my flat. I want a letter to the Council to help us move.'
'Someone is moving our furniture around the flat when we are not there, and at night when we are asleep.'
'I don't know who it is, but they are clever because they avoid all the traps I leave for them. Locks are no problem to them.'
'They are going to harm John (husband) and me, I just know it.'
'I can't sleep. Could you with people calling you names all night?'
'Names like "slut" and "bitch".'
'Two voices always talking about me, telling me that I'm worthless.'
'It must be the neighbours, they are interfering with my head making me

do things. Yes, like telling me to jump out of the window. They are controlling my legs.'
'They know when I go out because they can read my mind.'
'I'm not ill you know, I just need a new flat. All my problems would be over if I had a new flat.'
'I don't want to die, I never considered killing myself, but the neighbours want me dead.'

There was no obvious impairment of consciousness, and she was orientated in time, place and person.
Physical examination was normal.

Questions

1 What abnormalities of this woman's mental state are evident from the history?
2 What is the diagnosis?
3 How do you differentiate an organic from a functional psychosis?
4 Which section of the Mental Health Act (1983) would you use to detain this patient if she attempted to leave the department?

Answers

1 Abnormalities in her mental state are:

Appearance and behaviour: she appeared anxious and agitated. The constant furtive glances (hypervigilance) towards the door suggest that she is suspicious.

Thoughts: normal structure of thinking. No formal thought disorder.

Delusional ideas: persecutory delusions – she believed that persons were moving the furniture around and were trying to harm her.
Thought interference – her neighbours knew when she was going out because they could read her mind.

Perception: disorder of perception – she experienced the auditory hallucination of hearing voices which were addressing her and saying derogatory things about her such as 'you are worthless'. These are second person auditory hallucinations.

Passivity: feelings of passivity – she felt her legs were controlled by her neighbours.

Insight: degree of insight into the illness – her insight was poor. She actually stated that she was not ill, and that everything would be alright if only they had a new flat.

2 The putative diagnosis is an acute paranoid psychosis.

This would appear to be her first episode of a psychosis, and she needs admission because:

- there is a potential risk of self-harm, and
- to allow a longitudinal assessment of this illness.

Potential underlying conditions which might have precipitated this acute event include:

a *Organic state*
   i Acute – drug intoxication or withdrawal, infection etc.
   ii dementia
b Affective disorder – underlying manic-depressive illness.
c Schizophrenia.
d Schizo-affective and other atypical psychoses, e.g. psychogenic, that is overwhelming stress, e.g. two or three major life events occurring in close succession.

The most important of these to consider particularly in a patient with a first episode of a psychotic illness is an acute organic state which may present as a functional psychosis.

3 It is usually not difficult to distinguish between an organic and functional state. However, on occasion real difficulties do arise, and the misdiagnosis particularly of an acute organic state can be fatal. There are many conditions which may give rise to an acute organic state (for a list of some common causes see p. 202).

The most important clinical features which suggest an organic rather than a function state are *clouding of consciousness* and *disorientation in time and place.*

Impairment of consciousness may be absent when you first see the patient as it tends to fluctuate throughout the day, typically being worse at night (sundowning). Mild impairment of consciousness may be subtle and manifest as inattention rather than drowsiness.

Additional history from a relative or friend can be invaluable here as they may have noticed the periodic nature of the impairment. Episodes of delirium may be punctuated by periods of clear thought. In addition, there is global impairment of cognitive processes and a reduced awareness of the environment.

Associated disorders of thinking and perception are common. These give rise to delusional ideas (often persecutory), ideas of reference, which are poorly developed and rarely sustained and hallucinations which are typically visual but may be auditory or tactile. It is these features, delusions and hallucinations which, when present, are most likely to give the impression that the patient has a functional condition.

Any physical symptoms complained of should always be taken seriously and a full medical history (if available) and clinical examination is necessary in all patients.

Hypoglycaemia, infection, metabolic disorders, alcohol and drug abuse all need to be actively excluded. Any patient with a potential organic illness should be assessed by the medical team before seeing the psychiatrist.

4 This woman needs admission to hospital for assessment, investigation and treatment. She is at risk of causing harm to herself, acting on instructions from the auditory hallucinations. She should be referred to the duty psychiatrist for assessment and admission. If she is unwilling to consent to informal admission to hospital then she should be detained under the relevant section of the Mental Health Act (1983). There are two Sections of this Act enabling the patient to be detained which are relevant to work in the Accident and Emergency department.

A *Section 2 (assessment order)*: this is the most commonly used section of the Act for acutely ill patients who present to the emergency services. It allows the patient to be detained for up to 28 days for assessment, followed if necessary by treatment. To complete this Section requires the signatures of two doctors, one of whom must be approved under Section 12 of the Act (a senior registrar or consultant psychiatrist), and either the signature of an approved local authority social worker, or the nearest relative (the relative should be used as a last resort as their signature may be the source of bitter resentment in the future).

To satisfy the conditions of the Act the patient must fulfil the following criteria:

1 Be suffering from a mental disorder (the specific type of disorder is not specified and is open to interpretation)
2 Unwilling to be admitted to hospital
3 Requires admission either for their own health and safety, or the protection of others.

B *Section 4 (emergency order)*: this Section should only be used in an emergency if an approved psychiatrist is not available. It allows the patient to be detained for up to 72 h for assessment only. The signature of *any* post-registration doctor is required along with that of either the closest relative or approved local authority social worker. Once the patient is detained in hospital under this Section it is normally converted to a Section 2 as soon as it is feasible to do so.

When the decision to admit a mentally ill patient has been made you should clearly inform them of the proposal and explain what this will entail (as you would do when admitting a patient with an organic illness). If the patient is unhappy with this suggestion, positive reinforcement from relatives and friends may be helpful.

If the patient cannot be persuaded to stay as an informal patient then she should be detained using the relevant Section. This can be a time-consuming process and it may be difficult to detain the patient while waiting for the relevant papers to be completed. If the patient does attempt to leave during this period and there are compelling reasons to believe that the patient is at risk of harming herself or others by allowing her to leave you should restrain them under common law.

This may be impossible, and if the patient does leave then there is little you can do. The police should be informed and will often attempt to return the patient if she can be found. The general practitioner also has to be informed as he may be the next doctor to see the patient.

If the patient has expressed thoughts of harming particular persons (e.g. husband) then if possible they should be contacted and informed of the developments. Some care needs to be exercised over what information is passed on to these people, as divulging personal medical information may compromise the confidentiality of the doctor–patient relationship. The degree of danger that these people are thought to be in will determine what is said.

Careful documentation of the whole episode is necessary.

Note: In addition to these two Sections you should be aware of Section 136.

Section 136 (place of safety order): the police are able to detain in a place of safety an individual thought to be mentally ill, who is displaying disturbing abnormal behaviour in a public place. This Section enables the person to be detained for assessment only for up to 72 h and requires the signature of one police constable. The place of safety may be the police station or a designated accident department or psychiatric ward.

When the accident department is the designated place of safety in the district the police should remain in attendance until the duty psychiatrist and, ideally, the duty social worker have assessed the patient. If the patient is indeed mentally ill and requires admission then the Section 136 is changed to Section 2. If the patient leaves before the assessment is complete then the Section 136 is still in force and it is the responsibility of the police to find and return the person.

If the person is considered not to be suffering from a mental illness and the police do not wish to charge them, then they may be discharged. All such persons should be seen by the duty social worker.

Reference

Goldberg, D., Benjamin, S. and Creed, F. (1987) *Psychiatry in Medical Practice.* Tavistock Publications, London

Case 23

A 37-year-old man suddenly became aggressive and confused during a business meeting and had to be restrained by his colleagues. They noted him to be sweaty, pale and cold to touch. An ambulance was called, and on arrival in the Accident and Emergency department he was still combative but quite drowsy and continually yawning.

Question

What is the diagnosis to exclude?

Answer

The diagnosis to exclude in this man is hypoglycaemia. This condition is most commonly the result of too much exogenous insulin, or oral hypoglycaemic agents. It can give rise to a variety of symptoms, such as bizarre behaviour, aggression, irritability and appearing drunk. The signs are confusion, altered consciousness, pallor, sweating, palpitations and yawning.

It is easily reversed with either 50 ml of 50% glucose as an i.v. bolus, or i.m. glucagon when venous access is a problem.

There are many other conditions which may present with an acute confusional state (see Case 59) but none so readily treatable as hypoglycaemia.

Case 24

A 15-year-old boy came home from school at 16:00 and complained to his mother that he had a headache. His mother was concerned, as this was an unusual complaint in her son, but more particularly so because there had been an 'outbreak' of meningitis in the school 6 weeks previously. She learnt from her son that the headache developed after a game of football. During the game he had collided with another boy, and they had hit their heads together, but neither of them had thought twice about it. While taking his temperature, the boy vomited. This prompted the mother to ring the general practitioner requesting a visit. While waiting, it was apparent that the boy was becoming progressively incoherent, confused and drowsy. She then called for an ambulance. On arrival at hospital the boy was vomiting, confused and apathetic. Apart from seasonal rhinitis there was no other significant medical history.

On examination:

- Airway clear
- Respiratory rate 12/min, normal pattern
- Chest clear
- Blood pressure 150/85 mmHg, pulse 68/min
- Abdomen soft, bowel sounds normal
- Head – no evidence of injury
- Eye opening to verbal command
- Confused speech

- Obeyed commands and moved all four limbs appropriately
- Pupils unequal in size, right 5 mm, left 3 mm
- Direct response to light was sluggish in the right, but normal in the left
- Doll's head movements normal
- Oculovestibular normal
- Corneal reflex present
- Gag reflexes intact
- Motor – evidence of mild (4/5) left-sided weakness with an extensor plantar response

The boy then had a tonic-clonic seizure lasting 45 s–1 min, which terminated spontaneously without the use of drugs.

Questions

1 What is the emergency management?
2 What is the Glasgow coma score?
3 What is the diagnosis?

Answers

1 See Appendix

2 Glasgow coma score

Glasgow coma score is 12.

3 Diagnosis

This young man presented with a deteriorating level of consciousness with a dilating right pupil which was sluggish in its response to light and a contralateral weakness. These features are very suggestive of an expanding supratentorial mass compressing the brainstem laterally. This is known as the uncal syndrome. In this clinical setting an extradural haematoma is the most likely diagnosis. The immediate management therefore consists of intubating and ventilating the patient after sedation, organizing a CT scan and contacting the neurosurgeons.

An expanding lesion in the lateral middle fossa or temporal lobe pushes the uncus and hippocampal gyrus over the free lateral edge of the tentorium. The earliest consistent sign of this herniation is a unilateral dilating pupil which is sluggish in response to light and occurs on the same side as the lesion. Motor signs may be difficult to elicit but usually consist of mild contralateral weakness.

Deterioration, if it occurs, tends to be rapid after this stage, as the brainstem becomes progressively disturbed. The pupil dilates fully and becomes unresponsive and the oculocephalic response reveals oculomotor involvement with loss of movement of the affected eye. Ipsilateral weakness may then develop due to pressure exerted on the cerebral peduncles by the contralateral edge of the tentorium. The respiratory pattern, though initially normal, may change to sustained hyperventilation.

Finally, there is a full-blown third nerve palsy, absent brainstem reflexes and decorticate or decerebrate posturing of the limbs.

Extradural haematomas typically are said to produce a period of primary unconsciousness then a lucid period, followed by progressive deterioration. However, only approximately 20% of patients actually adhere to this sequence. Studies have pointed to the fact that extradural haematomas may develop in patients who never lost consciousness at the time of injury, and who regarded their injury as too trivial to warrant hospital attention. In these patients headache, irritability, drowsiness and vomiting are the usual clear signs of impending trouble. Approximately 15% of patients will have no skull fracture. Pupillary signs are the most useful early indicator and should be assessed thoroughly.

The mortality rate increases dramatically by the time the pupil becomes fixed and dilated.

Outcome

This young man had an extradural haematoma demonstrated on CT scan and after evacuation made an uneventful recovery.

References

Plum, F. and Posner, J. B. (1980) *The Diagnosis of Stupor and Coma.* (3rd edn) F. A. Davis Co., Philadelphia

Springings, D. and Chambers, J. (1990) *Acute Medicine.* Blackwell Scientific Publications, Oxford

Case 25

A 12-year-old girl fell over on the pavement and knocked out her left upper incisor. She had badly bruised her upper lip but there was no other apparent injury. Her mother brought the tooth with her.

Question

What is your management?

Answer

When a patient completely avulses an incisor tooth attempts should be made to re-implant it. The viability of an avulsed tooth deteriorates within an hour of being out of the socket.

The avulsed tooth should be cleaned in saline and gently inserted back into the socket. The reinsertion is usually readily achieved by the patients themselves. Once inserted it has to be held there. Numerous methods of securing it in place have been described. These include the use of chewing gum, aluminium foil, and tissue glue. If it proves impossible to reinsert the tooth then it should be stored either in milk, or the patient can carry it in her own buccal sulcus (not suitable for children).

All patients should be referred urgently to the dentist. Ampicillin has been shown to improve the prognosis of re-implantation by controlling bacterial invasion of the tooth socket. In addition, 2% chlorhexidine mouth washes should be suggested, and the patient prescribed tetanus toxoid if necessary.

Further notes

More commonly than complete avulsion, teeth are chipped and broken. These injuries are associated with damage to the lips and gums.

Remember in these cases, and in cases of tooth avulsion when the tooth is not found, that fragments may have been inhaled, or contained within the upper lip.

Radiographs of the chest, and a soft tissue film of the upper lip, can reveal some very unexpected results.

Reference

Scheer, B. (1990) Emergency treatment of avulsed incisor teeth. Editorial. *British Medical Journal*, **301**,

Case 26

A 10-month-old baby boy was brought to the Accident and Emergency department by his father with diarrhoea and vomiting. Three days previously he had had a cough, runny nose and a fever. He had not been particularly unwell and had continued to feed well until the day before when he began vomiting. For 24 h he had been unable to keep even clear fluids down and had lost interest in his bottles. For the last 12 h he had had frequent watery, green stool and had had at least 10 nappy changes. The baby was irritable and cried a lot.

He had been born at term after an uneventful pregnancy and previously has been well apart from a similar episode of diarrhoea and vomiting 3 months previously. This episode had been mild and short lived. He had been initially breastfed for 2 months, but these were then changed for SMA Goldcap. Baby foods were introduced at 4 months and he was now on a mixed diet. Immunizations were up to date and he could now walk having sat at 7 months and could say 'mama, dada'. The family were living in temporary accommodation awaiting rehousing. Neither parent was working, but both were in good health.

On examination:

- Pyrexial 37.8°C
- Irritable, pale
- Respiratory rate 40/min
- Chest clear
- Pulse 130/min, warm peripheries
- Ears normal
- Mouth dry, red and encrusted secretions in nose and throat
- Fontanelle depressed
- Skin turgor – decreased elasticity
- Abdomen soft
- Bowel sounds normal
- Weight 7.3 kg

Questions

1 What is the most likely diagnosis?
2 What are the clinical signs of dehydration in a child?
3 What is your management in this case?
4 How would you advise the parents nursing a child at home with gastroenteritis?

Answers

1 The most likely diagnosis in this case is acute gastroenteritis complicated by a degree of dehydration. The commonest pathogen implicated in children is the rotavirus. The clinical presentation of viral gastroenteritis is very variable. Some children appear unaffected by their illness whereas others tolerate it very poorly. A low grade fever, vomiting and coryzal symptoms are variable features.

Bacterial gastroenteritis gives rise to a more systemic illness, with a high fever, irritability and bloody mucoid stools. Commonly implicated pathogens are *Salmonella, Shigella, E. coli* and *Campylobacter*.

Alternative diagnoses should include systemic infections which may be accompanied by gastrointestinal symptoms of diarrhoea and vomiting, particularly otitis media, pneumonia, meningitis and, in particular, urinary tract infection. Examination of the urine is commonly forgotten and should be included in the examination of all infants who are unwell.

Occasionally surgical diseases of intussusception and appendicitis may present in this fashion.

2 The early signs of dehydration can be very subtle, particularly in obese infants. It is always wise to err on the side of caution particularly if the history suggests significant fluid losses through the diarrhoea and vomiting, and fluid replacement (feeding) has been inadequate. Below are the clinical signs of dehydration.

Body weight lost (%)	Signs
<5	Child not well, dry mucous membranes, usually keen to feed
5–10	Apathetic, listless, unwell. Decreased skin turgor, sunken eyes and fontanelle, tachypnoea. Marked reduction in wet nappies
>10	Shocked, cold peripheries, hypotension, mottled cyanosed. Child obviously very unwell.
This is an emergency	Call paediatricians. Immediate resuscitation with intravenous fluid (20 ml/kg) is necessary

All children with clinically detectable dehydration should be referred for admission to hospital, as should children who may not appear dehydrated, but are likely to become so because oral replacement cannot keep up with losses, i.e. when a child is vomiting repeatedly or will not take oral fluids at all.

3 This child has the clinical signs of approximately 5% dehydration and should be referred to the paediatric team.

4 Children and infants who are well, without signs of dehydration or underlying systemic infection, may be managed at home under the supervision of the general practitioner. The parents should be advised to stop all milk and solids (though breast feeding should continue) for 24 h and replace them with an oral glucose and electrolyte mixture.

Adequate sachets of an approved proprietary brand (Rehidrat, Dioralyte) should be supplied and the parent instructed on how exactly to prepare them. The daily requirements are calculated from the weight of the child with the addition of 20% to cover continuing losses (see below). Half the calculated daily requirements should be given in the first 8 h as hourly feeds.

After 24 h, bottlefed babies can be restarted on their normal milk. If on restarting the feeds the diarrhoea worsens then the process should be repeated with 24 h of glucose and electrolyte mixture, and then regrading more slowly with 1/4 strength feeds for the next 24 h, then 1/2 strength etc. over the next few days.

Children failing to respond should be reviewed within 24 h, by the general practitioner. Any child brought back to the department with continuing symptoms should be discussed with and assessed by the paediatric team.

Daily glucose and electrolyte mixture requirement

Age	Weight (kg)	Mixtures (ml/kg)
Less than 6 months	Up to 5	150
6 months–1 year	5–10	120
1–3 years	10–15	100

Outcome

This child was nursed on the ward for 48 h. Small, regular feeds were given, which were well tolerated over the first day. The child's condition improved and the diarrhoea had settled within 36 h. Regular paracetamol was prescribed for the fever and the child was allowed home with instruction to return if the symptoms returned.

Practice points

1 Gastroenteritis is very common in children.
2 A thorough clinical assessment is necessary to exclude underlying pathology, and overt dehydration.
3 A full explanation to the parents is necessary to ensure correct management of fluid replacement at home.

A further 20% should be added to the total volume given in 24 h to cover additional losses, due to fever, vomiting and diarrhoea.

Reference

Salim, A. F. M. and Farthing, M. J. G. (1989) Acute diarrhoea in childhood. *Update*, 1 November, 787

Case 27

A 48-year-old woman had oysters at a business lunch. Thirty minutes later she developed crampy abdominal pain and profuse vomiting. She also noticed her hands had become swollen and had an intensely itchy rash on her upper trunk. She felt vertiginous every time she stood, and therefore had to sit while she vomited. During a protracted episode of vomiting she suddenly became limp and slipped to the ground. She was unresponsive for about 20 s, and then slowly regained consciousness. She felt better lying on the floor, but worse every time she attempted to rise from the supine position. An ambulance was called. Her past medical history included two episodes of iritis and a peptic ulcer for which she took cimetidine 800 mg at night. She had been taking the combined oral contraceptive pill as hormone replacement therapy for the last 2 years.

On examination:

- Very pale and sweaty
- Apyrexial
- Warm peripheries with a bounding good volume
- Pulse rate 110/min, blood pressure 70/40 mmHg lying
- She fainted every time she sat up
- Mouth, tongue and pharynx normal
- Respiratory rate 16/min
- Chest clear, no stridor, no wheeze, peak flow 410 l/min
- Abdomen soft
- Rectal examination – light brown liquid stool
- Skin – blotchy, urticarial and erythematous rash on upper trunk, shoulders and face, with swelling of eye lids and both hands
- While lying flat, she was lucid and conscious, no meningism, no focal signs

Questions

1 What is the diagnosis?
2 What is the treatment?

Answers

1 Diagnosis

The most likely diagnosis is anaphylactic shock. Alternative diagnoses that should be considered are acute gastrointestinal haemorrhage, or acute gastritis related to a toxin-producing organism. The clinical findings of a good volume bounding pulse would argue against hypovolaemia, and acute infective gastritis (e.g. staphylococcal) would normally be expected to take several hours to develop.

Anaphylactic shock

The term anaphylaxis is used to denote a generalized allergic reaction which is immunologically mediated and can give rise to life-threatening clinical manifestations. The most characteristic feature of anaphylaxis is its rapid onset after the administration of the antigen, which rapidly combines with a specific antibody resulting in the release of chemical mediators including histamine. In general the quicker the symptoms develop after exposure to the antigen the more severe the reaction. Anaphylaxis can develop within seconds of a parenterally administered antigen, and will usually develop within 30–45 min when the antigen is ingested.

The clinical manifestations are variable, depending to some extent upon the antigen, the route of exposure, and whether there is a family history of atopy.

Clinical manifestations are usually confined to: the skin, respiratory tract, gastrointestinal tract and the cardiovascular system. Typical symptoms are shown in Table 4.

Table 4   Typical symptoms of anaphylactic shock

Skin manifestations
    Diffuse erythema
    Urticaria
    Pruritis
    Oedema
    Sweating

Respiratory manifestations
    Laryngeal oedema
        Dyspnoea
        Hoarseness
        Stridor
        Dysphagia
    Bronchial mucosa
        Chest tightness
        Wheezing
        Cough
        Respiratory failure

Gastrointestinal tract
    Vomiting
    Diarrhoea
    Faecal or urinary incontinence
    Abdominal cramps

Cardiovascular system
    Tachycardia
    Hypotension
    Arrhythmias
    Atrial fibrillation
    Nodal rhythm
    ST, T wave changes

Making the diagnosis of anaphylaxis

As in this case, when symptoms develop within 30 min of exposure to an antigen known to precipitate anaphylaxis, such as shell fish, the diagnosis is straightforward, however, this is not always so.

Cautionary tale
A young man presented with acute severe asthma of sudden onset. He was known to be asthmatic. Despite oxygen and a bronchodilator he became progressively more distressed, cyanosed, and had a respiratory arrest. There was no evidence of a pneumothorax. He was intubated and adrenaline was given. Within 25 min he had extubated himself, he was alert and orientated, and had a peak flow of 420 l/min. He was now able to give a history that he had eaten a salad containing walnuts 30 min before the episode had started. A similar but much milder attack of wheezing had occurred the last time he did this.

With subsequent exposures symptoms usually become progressively severe, but do not necessarily give rise to the same clinical manifestations.

Cautionary tale
A 48-year-old man presented with progressive shortness of breath, stridor and a feeling of suffocation which had developed 20 min after taking two penicillin tablets. The penicillin had been prescribed for a sore throat. Adrenaline was given, and when intubated it was noted that his uveal and supraglottic structures were very swollen. He responded well to therapy and was extubated at 16 h. He recalled that this had not occurred the last time he was given penicillin, and he had never been told that he was allergic to it. Expanding on the past history, he had been given penicillin during a flu epidemic when he had a persistent productive cough. He had been unable to take many of the tablets because shortly after the first dose he got severe abdominal cramps, vomiting and profuse watery diarrhoea. The episode lasted 12 h and settled spontaneously. This had been put down to acute food poisoning as he had eaten a take away meal the night before.

Anaphylaxis should be considered in any patient who presents in shock.

Common antigens

Penicillin and insect stings (bee, wasp, hornet) are the commonest antigens to precipitate anaphylaxis in this country. However, a whole range of antigens has been documented producing anaphylaxis (Table 5).

2 Treatment

Adrenaline given by either subcutaneous or intramuscular injection is the treatment of choice, and is necessary in all cases when there is a generalized systemic reaction. Intravenous adrenaline should be given when there is respiratory arrest or cardiovascular collapse. The dose is

Table 5 Commonest antigens to precipitate anaphylaxis

Hormones
ACTH
Insulin
Hydrocortisone
Methylprednisolone

Food (by ingestion)
Shellfish
Nuts
Banana
Egg
Tuna

Antibiotics
Penicillins
Cephalosporin
Tetracyclines
Nitrofurantoin

Venom singing insects
Wasp
Bee
Hornet

Other drugs Aspirin Indomethacin Naproxen Ibuprofen Diagnostic agents Iodinated contrast media (Used in IVUs etc)	Although these drugs/agents produce a clinical picture indistinguishable from acute anaphylaxis, these are probably not caused by immunological mediated reactions, and are therefore called anaphylactoid reactions. The treatment, however, is exactly the same.

0.5–1 ml of 1:1000 adrenaline (0.5–1 mg) or 5–10 ml of 1:10 000 adrenaline (0.5–1 mg). This should be repeated every 5–15 min depending on its response until there has been clinical improvement.

General management includes preservation of vital functions with emphasis on the **airway**, **breathing** and **circulation**.

Airway and breathing. All patients should be given 60% oxygen. For patients with symptoms (tightness in the throat) or signs of impending respiratory distress, hoarseness, stridor, oedema of the tongue or uvula, adrenaline should be given and the anaesthetist called immediately.

Patients with overt respiratory distress will need intubation, or if this is not possible because of the oedema, a surgical airway (needle or surgical cricothyroidotomy) is necessary.

Wheeze, dyspnoea and chest tightness should be treated with adrenaline i.m./s.c. and by nebulized bronchodilator.

Circulation. For circulatory arrest, full basic life support is necessary and adrenaline given intravenously. This should be repeated every 5 min until the circulation is restored, and the patient resuscitated using the guidelines suggested by the Resuscitation Council (UK).

Patients with a systolic blood pressure of greater than 90 mmHg should be placed in the head down position, and adrenaline given i.m./s.c.

For patients with a systolic blood pressure of less than 90 mmHg, i.m./s.c. adrenaline should be given, and infusion of 500 ml of colloid commenced. Repeat of adrenaline every 5–15 min, and continued fluid administration is necessary until the perfusion pressure is restored.

For elderly patients and those with known impaired cardiac performance, central pressure monitoring will be necessary.

The occasional patient will need inotropic support.

Additional therapy

1 Local infiltration of adrenaline into the site of the sting or injection may help to slow absorption; 2–3 ml of 1:10 000 only should be used for this purpose.
2 Intravenous chlorpheniramine 10 mg.
3 Intravenous hydrocortisone 200 mg.
4 Nebulized bronchodilator to relieve bronchoconstriction.

Response to treatment is variable. Some patients make a dramatic recovery, others will need intensive therapy for up to 24 h. Patients who respond well should be observed for 4 h, and if asymptomatic after this period can be discharged.

The antigen responsible for the episode should be identified and avoidance of further exposure discussed with the patient. For patients in whom further exposure cannot be prevented, mini-adrenaline ampoules, or adrenaline inhalers are available to be taken at times of further exposure. The general practitioner should be informed directly of the episode and the most likely antigen involved.

Outcome

This woman responded quickly to adrenaline 0.5 mg s.c. and 500 ml of colloid. Within 4 h she was asymptomatic with a normal blood pressure and wanted to go home. She was given a letter to her general practitioner detailing the episode and advised to abstain from eating shell fish in the future.

Reference

Springings, D. and Chambers, J. (1990) *Acute Medicine.* Blackwell Scientific Publishers, Oxford

Case 28

An 86-year-old woman was brought to the Accident and Emergency department with a letter from the warden of her flat.

Dear Doctor,
Re: Amy Jackson, DOB 4.3.1904
I found this lady on the floor by the kitchen in her flat this morning. Her bed had not been slept in and I fear she has been on the floor all night. She is normally independent, mobile and sound of mind, though this morning she was rather vague. She is capable of shopping for herself and normally walks with the aid of a stick. She is quite deaf and refuses to wear her hearing aid. Her daughter normally comes to see her once a week though she has not been for the past three weeks. She has been well recently, although she had a heart attack five years ago.
Medication:
 Panadol
 Ponstan
 Frumil
 Lanoxin
 Mogadon

Yours
M S Smith
Home Warden

On examination:

- Temperature 35.8°C
- Not orientated in time, place or person
- Unable to give any further coherent history
- Mental test score 2/10
- Tongue dry, skin turgor decreased, cold peripheries
- Respiratory rate 20/min
- Not cyanosed, no obvious respiratory distress. Bilateral basal crepitations
- Pulse 106/min regular, blood pressure 90/60 mmHg
- Heart sounds – aortic systolic murmur
- Abdomen soft, no masses
- Rectal examination – constipated
- Tender right hip with limited passive range of movement
- No obvious head injury, no neck stiffness
- Formal neurological testing was difficult due to poor compliance though there were no obvious focal neurological signs. Both plantars were down going.

Question

What is your management of the elderly patient who presents having been found on the floor?

Answer

Falls in the elderly are common, and undoubtedly some are simply accidental in nature due to factors such as poor mobility and visual impairment. However, in common with other common presenting complaints, such as 'unable to cope', 'won't get out of bed', 'off her legs', and confusion, falls may be indicative of an acute underlying condition.

There are two basic principles that you should always bear in mind when assessing the elderly:

i Non-specific presentations of acute illness are common in the elderly
ii Multiple pathology is common.

The history of the presenting illness is commonly incomplete, and there is no substitute for contacting relatives, friends or the general practitioner for any additional history.

A social history should also be obtained. Form an impression of what they normally can do for themselves, what support they have, (relatives?, district nurse?, meals on wheels?) and what additional support they may require if they are to be discharged home.

Clinical examination can be remarkably misleading with few convincing physical signs even in the presence of serious pathology, e.g. lack of peritonism with a perforated viscus, or lack of a fever in the presence of a septicaemia. Examination should always include an assessment of the patient's mental state (mental test score see p. 204) and their mobility. Patients living alone, and unable to transfer from bed to chair at the very least, will be unable to cope without constant home support. The aim of investigations should be to exclude conditions which commonly gives rise to sudden deterioration in the elderly. These include:

- Infections – urine, chest
- Congestive cardiac failure
- Silent ischaemia, arrhythmias
- Dehydration, postural hypotension
- Drug side effects, drug overdose
- Hypothermia
- Stroke/transient ischaemic attack

Base line investigations should include:

- Full blood count
- Measure the temperature with a low reading thermometer if hypothermia is suspected
- Blood cultures
- Glucose (initial BM stix estimation)
- Urea and electrolytes
- Electrocardiogram
- Chest radiograph
- Other radiographs as directed by clinical examination
- One should have a low threshold for X-raying the hips and the skull

Outcome

This woman presented with a fall and is found to be acutely confused. The initial differential diagnosis included infection, myocardial infarction, dehydration secondary to diuretics, or a possible drug overdose. In addition a possible fracture of the neck of femur had to be excluded. Initial investigations revealed no evidence of an acute myocardial event, though she was dehydrated with raised urea. Chest radiograph demonstrated no acute lung pathology or cardiac failure, and two views of the right hip did not reveal an obvious fracture of the femur, though there was a fracture of the inferior pubis ramus on the right.

She was referred to the care of the elderly team. The ultimate diagnosis was septicaemia secondary to a urinary tract infection.

Case 29

A 39-year-old man presented with persistent epistaxis for 2 h. He had recently had a cold, and since that time had been subject to intermittent nose bleeds.

Question

What is your management?

Answer

Epistaxis is described as being either anterior or posterior depending upon the site of the bleeding. Generally speaking children bleed from the congested mucosa on the nasal septum visible at the front of the nose (Little's area), and elderly patients tend to bleed from the arteriosclerotic blood vessels situated more posteriorly. Anterior bleeding is commonly precipitated by nose picking. It is relatively easy to manage as the site of haemorrhage is accessible to digital compression and cautery. By contrast posterior bleeds are inaccessible and can pose a serious management problem.

When there appears to be bilateral bleeding from the nose, this usually due to the blood tracking around the nasal septum posteriorly rather than a separate site in each nostril. The side where the bleeding was first noticed should be assumed to contain the source.

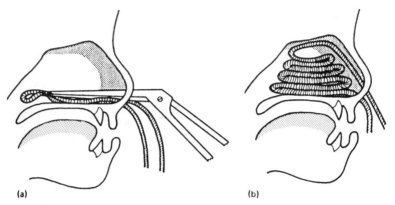

(a)   (b)

Figure 7 (a) Anterior nasal packing introducing the first loop along the floor of the nose and building upwards. (b) The pack in place (From Brown, A. F. T. (1992) *Accident and Emergency: Diagnosis and Management.* 2nd edn. Butterworth-Heinemann, Oxford)

The management of epistaxis

1 *Assess the cardiovascular status of the patient.* Elderly patients in particular are prone to severe nose bleeds with significant blood loss, especially if they are on anticoagulants. Occasionally, initial resuscitation of the patient with intravenous fluids and blood is necessary.

2 *Institute simple first aid measures.* Sit the patient down, head forward, and instruct him on how to pinch the anterior cartilaginous part of the nose between his index finger and thumb. Provide a bowl for him to spit out any blood running down his throat, rather than swallowing it.

Emphasize the necessity for constant pressure for 5 min. This will terminate most anterior bleeds. If it does not, repeat the pressure having first inserted a small pledget of cotton wool up the nostril which has been soaked in 0.5 ml of 1:10 000 adrenaline (not in the elderly). Alternatively cocaine paste may be used.

3 *Cauterize any anterior bleeding point.* Cautery with silver nitrate sticks is effective. Having terminated the bleeding, and anaesthetized the nose with cocaine paste apply the silver nitrate for 40 s to the most likely bleeding point. To prevent a caustic burn to the upper lip, Vaseline should be applied prior to cautery. Electrocautery, if available, is an alternative. Only one side of the septum should be cauterized, otherwise necrosis and perforation may ensue.

If an obvious anterior bleeding site is not seen, or in the unusual case of not being able to control anterior bleeding nasal packing should follow.

4 *Nasal packs.* The nose is packed with 1 inch (2.5 cm) ribbon gauze, which is impregnated with either bismuth and iodoform paraffin paste (BIPP) or Vaseline. It is a very uncomfortable procedure and adequate local anaesthetic is necessary. With a good light and angled forceps (Tilley's) the ribbon gauze is packed in the nose in a zig-zag fashion starting on the nasal floor and moving towards the roof. Both ends of the pack should be left out of the nose and secured with a safety pin. It is usual to pack both nostrils, though some authors advocate that only one is necessary. As inhalation of the pack is a possibility, it is current practice in many departments to admit patients when a nasal pack has been inserted. If you are unfamiliar with the packing of a nose, or it fails to control the haemorrhage, then you should seek the advice of your consultant or the ENT surgeon.

5 *Nasal balloons.* If a nasal pack has not successfully controlled the haemorrhage then a nasal balloon is an alternative method of haemorrhage control. There are some balloons available which are specifically manufactured for the job (Brighton). A foley catheter (14F, 16F) is a readily available and much cheaper alternative. The catheter is run along the floor of the nostril, and down into the post-nasal space until the tip can be seen in the pharynx. The balloon is then inflated with 5–10 ml of air, and withdrawn until resistance is felt. Traction should not be exerted on the catheter, as it is there to stop the blood escaping posteriorly, rather than to provide local tamponade. The anterior nose is then packed with ribbon gauze. On occasions a post nasal pack, or rarely surgery is necessary to control the bleeding.

Outcome

This man did not have an obvious anterior bleeding site, and digital pressure did not control the epistaxis. Nasal packing did however, and he was admitted under the care of the ENT surgeons.

Reference

Brown, A. F. T. (1992) *Accident and Emergency: Diagnosis and Management.* 2nd edn. Butterworth-Heinemann, Oxford
Browning, G. G. (1987) *Updated ENT.* 2nd edn. Butterworths, London

Case 30

On the way to work one morning, you notice in the road outside the hospital a group of people standing round an elderly man on the ground. A passer-by tells you that he suddenly collapsed as he was walking, and that an ambulance has been called. The man is lying on his back, appears to be in his sixties and looks lifeless.

Questions

1 What is your immediate management?
2 What factors determine a favourable outcome for this man?

An ambulance arrives and transports the patient to the Accident and Emergency department.

3 What are your priorities on arrival?
4 The monitor suggests your patient is in asystole. What is your management?

Answers

1 Immediate management

Your initial management at the scene should consist of:

Assessment: quickly assess the scene to ensure that while caring for this man, you are not putting your own life in danger. If he is actually on the road, instruct someone to stop the traffic etc. Having minimized the risk to yourself, gently shake him by the shoulders and ask 'Are you alright?' (Figure 8). If unresponsive move on to:

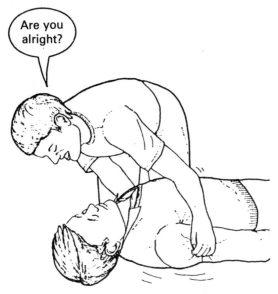

Figure 8 Establish consciousness (From Evans, T. R. (ed.) (1990) *ABC of Resuscitation*. BMJ Publications, London)

a **Airway**: look inside the mouth and remove any obstructing debris such as dislodged teeth or vomit with a sweep of the index finger around the oral cavity (Figure 9). Then maintain airway patency by performing a 'chin lift' manoeuvre (Figure 10). In the unconscious patient the tongue tends to flop back and obstruct the oropharynx and the 'chin lift' is designed to correct this. Having cleared and maintained the airway then ascertain whether or not he is breathing.

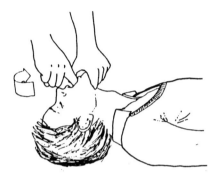

Figure 9 Finger sweeps (From Evans, T.R. (ed.) (1990) *ABC of Resuscitation*. BMJ Publications, London)

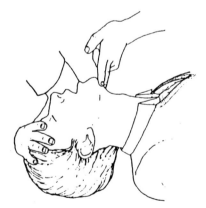

Figure 10 Head tilt and jaw lift (From Evans, T. R. (ed.) (1990) *ABC of Resuscitation*. BMJ Publications, London)

b **Breathing**: look, feel and listen. Look at the chest wall for respiratory excursions, while placing your cheek over the mouth, feeling and listening for breaths. It can be very difficult to be absolutely sure whether a person is breathing in some circumstances, for instance by the side of a busy road in the dark. If in doubt, assume spontaneous respiration is absent and commence mouth-to-mouth respirations.

Intermittent 'gasping' respirations are commonly present in a patient for several minutes after a cardiac arrest. These should be ignored as they will not provide adequate ventilation and the patient needs artificial ventilation.

Unresponsive patients with adequate ventilation (respiratory rate >10/min) should be placed in the recovery position and the ambulance awaited (Figure 11).

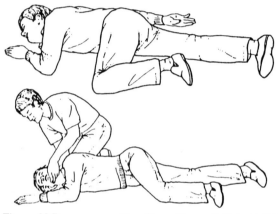

Figure 11 Recovery position (From Evans, T. R. (ed.) (1990) *ABC of Resuscitation*. BMJ Publications, London)

Mouth-to-mouth ventilation is performed in the following fashion.

While continuing to perform the 'chin lift', the other hand should pinch the nose and slightly extend the neck. Take a deep breath, form an airtight seal with your lips over the patient's. Forcibly exhale and watch for the chest wall to rise (Figure 12). If the chest wall does not rise with ventilation then you are being ineffective. Adjust your technique and try again. Perform two initial breaths, allowing the chest wall to deflate in between. Then assess the circulation.

c **Circulation**: feel for the carotid pulse (Figure 13). Allow 6 s before being convinced that it is absent. Then commence external cardiac massage. Place the heel of your hand two finger breadths above the xiphisternum, and place the other hand on top of the first (Figure 14). With your arms fully extended, and with your shoulders directly above your hands compress the chest in a rhythmical fashion counting 'one' and 'two' and 'three'... for 15 compressions. The rate of compressions should be sufficient to perform 80 compressions in 1 min.

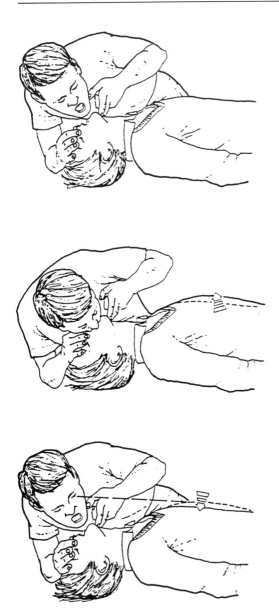

Figure 12 Expired air resuscitation (From Evans, T. R. (ed.) (1990) *ABC of Resuscitation*. BMJ Publications, London)

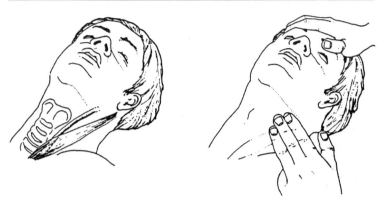

Figure 13 Check carotid pulse (From Evans, T. R. (ed.) (1990) *ABC of Resuscitation*. BMJ Publications, London)

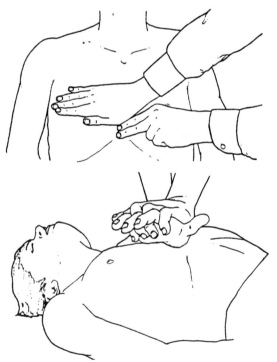

Figure 14 Position of hands for chest compression (From Evans, T. R. (ed.) (1990) *ABC of Resuscitation*. BMJ Publications, London)

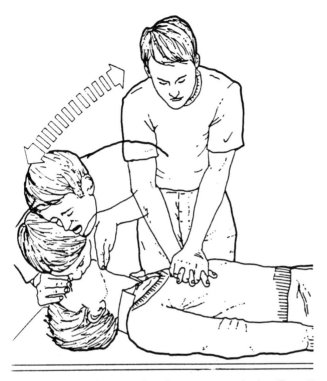

Figure 15 One rescuer cardiopulmonary resuscitation (From Evans, T. R. (ed.) (1990) *ABC of Resuscitation*. BMJ Publications, London)

The ratio of two breaths to 15 chest compressions should be continued if there is only one resuscitator (Figure 15). If there are two, one breath to every five chest compressions is the recommended ratio (Figure 16). Every 2 min the patient should be quickly reassessed for signs of spontaneous respiration or cardiac output. Otherwise basic life support should be continued at all times, now, in the ambulance, and in the Accident and Emergency department.

2 Factors determining a favourable outcome

Studies, most notably from Seattle, suggest that there are two factors that favourably alter the outcome of cardiac resuscitation in the community. These are (i) the speed with which basic life support is started, (ii) the time it takes to defibrillate the patient.

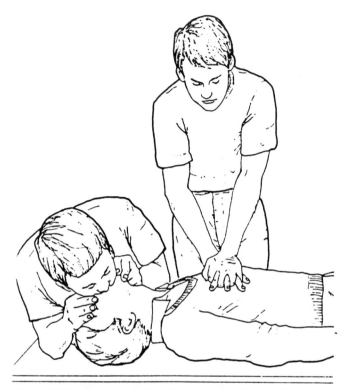

Figure 16 Two rescuer cardiopulmonary resuscitation (From Evans, T. R. (ed.) (1990) *ABC of Resuscitation*. BMJ Publications, London)

In Seattle an increasing percentage of patients are surviving resuscitation in the community, because as many as two-thirds of the local residents are trained in basic life support. In this country various community-based programmes are attempting to increase the success rate of resuscitation by training the general public. As a consequence we are seeing more patients in whom basic life support was commenced immediately. However, we still have a long way to go.

Cautionary tale
A 56-year-old man was dining at a restaurant with his wife. He suddenly felt unwell, and slumped forward with his face landing in his soup. Everyone was shocked and embarrassed as nobody knew what to do. The management called an ambulance and surrounded the man with a screen so that other patrons would not be upset. The ambulance arrived within 15 min and found the man dead, still with his face in the soup.

3 Priorities in hospital

The priorities on arrival in hospital are:

a Continue basic life support at all times. It should not be interrupted to perform any procedure for longer than 10 s.

b Immediately defibrillate the patient with 200 Joules.

c Intubate and ventilate with 100% oxygen, or if this is not possible ventilate with a bag and mask and supplemented oxygen.

d Connect the patient to a monitor, and treat the rhythm as appropriate.

e Achieve central venous access.

4 Management of asystole

Whenever a patient appears to be in asystole on a monitor always check that (a) the patient is correctly connected to the monitor and that it is working and (b) that the amplitude of the wave form is maximized by turning up the 'gain'. Fine ventricular fibrillation and asystole can be difficult to distinguish from one another. As the outcome from ventricular fibrillation is much superior to that of asystole always treat any debatable rhythm as ventricular fibrillation. Being satisfied that the patient is asystolic, management should be in accordance with the Resuscitation Council (UK) guidelines (Figure 17).

During the resuscitation of this patient sinus rhythm is produced with a rate of 100/min. However, this fails to produce an output.

Questions

5 What is this situation called?

6 What is your further management?

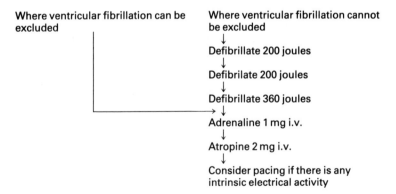

Where ventricular fibrillation can be excluded

Where ventricular fibrillation cannot be excluded
↓
Defibrillate 200 joules
↓
Defibrilate 200 joules
↓
Defibrillate 360 joules
→ ↓
Adrenaline 1 mg i.v.
↓
Atropine 2 mg i.v.
↓
Consider pacing if there is any intrinsic electrical activity

Figure 17 Algorithm for asystole (From Evans, T. R. (ed.) (1990) *ABC of Resuscitation*. BMJ Publications, London)

Answers

5 This situation, when the monitor demonstrates a good quality rhythm, but there is no output is termed electromechanical dissociation.

6 Following the recommendations of the Resuscitation Council (UK) the management is as follows:

Electromechanical dissociation
↓
Adrenaline 1 mg i.v.
↓
Consider specific therapy for
   pneumothorax
   hypovolaemia
   cardiac tamponade
   pulmonary embolus
↓
Consider calcium chloride (10 ml of 10%) for
   hyperkalaemia
   hypocalcaemia
   calcium antagonists

Notes on electromechanical dissociation

a Adrenaline 1 mg i.v., repeated every 5 min.
b Consider specific therapy for treatable conditions which may give rise to electromechanical dissociation, namely

   i *Tension pneumothorax*. By impeding venous return a tension pneumothorax can give rise to electromechanical dissociation. In the setting of a cardiac resuscitation both positive pressure ventilation, or external cardiac compression may give rise to this complication. If there is evidence of diminished air entry on one side of the chest, and evidence of tracheal deviation to the opposite side then a tension pneumothorax is likely. Immediate decompression is necessary. This can easily be performed by placing a cannula attached to a syringe in the second intercostal space in the midclavicular line. Easy aspiration of air confirms the diagnosis, the syringe should be removed and the cannula left in place. This having been done, the patient's condition should significantly improve. If no air is aspirated then remove the cannula. The risk of having created a pneumothorax now exists and should be considered throughout the remainder of the resuscitation.
     Beware: malposition of the endotracheal tube down the right main bronchus can lead to diminished breath sounds on the left.

ii *Hypovolaemia.* Acute hypovolaemia from, for example a ruptured aortic aneurysm, may give rise to electromechanical dissociation. A fluid bolus (1 l) given on an empirical basis may produce a femoral pulse. If the circulation is rapidly restored a surgeon should be called immediately.

iii *Cardiac tamponade.* This is uncommon in the absence of penetrating trauma, but can occur spontaneously secondary to a dissection of the aorta or rupture of the myocardium following a myocardial infarction. In any patient failing to respond to the measures above, aspiration of the myocardium should always be attempted. Using a 60 ml syringe attached to a long wide bore needle, enter the skin at an angle of 30° just to the left of the xiphisternum, and aim towards the tip of the left shoulder, aspirating as you advance the needle. When blood flushes back aspirate 100 ml. If tamponade is present this will lead to a clinical improvement. Knowing whether you are aspirating the pericardium or a ventricle in practice can be difficult. Practically, the best guide to indicate whether you are aspirating the heart is to watch the monitor during the procedure. The presence of ectopics or ST elevation in the existing complexes indicate when the ventricular muscle is being stimulated.

iv *Pulmonary embolus.* Without a thoracotomy this situation is rapidly fatal. In the postoperative patient, or a patient with a past history of an embolus, pulmonary embolus is a distinct possibility. Fragmentation of the obstructing embolus may occur during external cardiac massage so that it moves more peripherally and therefore does not produce such a profound haemodynamic effect. Streptokinase administered down a central line is a possible therapeutic option, however it is rarely successful in this situation.

v *Consider the use of calcium chloride.* Calcium chloride is no longer recommended for routine use in all cardiac arrest situations, but it may be helpful when electromechanical dissociation is secondary to hypocalcaemia, hyperkalaemia, or due to an overdose of calcium antagonists.

Practical points to remember during cardiac resuscitation

1 Central line administration of drugs is preferable to peripheral administrations. The femoral vein is a useful route to consider for primary access, rather than the neck as the operator can work without interfering with intubation, external cardiac massage, or removal of the clothes. The endotracheal administration of drugs should only be used if venous access is difficult to establish as it is much more difficult to achieve adequate serum levels by this route, even in double the standard dose. Adrenaline, lignocaine and atropine are all suitable for

Table 6 Drugs and dosages for cardiac arrest

Drug	Dose	Indications	Notes
Adrenaline	1 mg i.v. bolus	First line drug in asystole, ventricular fibrillation, electromechanical dissociation	Give as 10 ml of 1:10 000 rather than 1 ml of 1:1000. Repeat every 5 min
Atropine	2–2.4 mg i.v. bolus	Asystole	2.4 mg will achieve complete vagal block
	0.6–1.2 mg i.v. bolus	Bradyarrhythmias	
Lignocaine	100 mg i.v. bolus	Ventricular fibrillation	May be repeated to a total dose of 3 mg/kg. If successful start lignocaine infusion 4 mg/min reducing to 1 mg/min in 24 h
Sodium bicarbonate	50 ml of 8.4% i.v. slow bolus	Prolonged onset >15 min. Documented acidosis	Routine use is no longer recommended
Bretylium tosylate	500 mg (5–10 mg/kg) i.v. bolus	Resistant ventricular fibrillation	May take 20–30 min to be effective

administration down the endotracheal tube. *There is no role for intracardiac administration of drugs.*

2 Administer adrenaline 1 mg i.v. every 5 min in a prolonged arrest.

3 Allow at least 2 min for drugs to have an effect, because of the increase in circulation time.

4 The early use of sodium bicarbonate is no longer encouraged. In prolonged arrests (>15 min) 50 mmol of 8.4% sodium bicarbonate should be given on an empirical basis, otherwise it should only be given to correct a measured acidosis.

5 *Post-resuscitation care.* With the restoration of the circulation, the patient should be stabilized. The following are necessary:
   i Arterial blood gases: hypoxia, acid-base disturbance
   ii Urea and electrolytes: in particular to look for hypo-, or hyper-kalaemia
   iii Electrocardiogram: for evidence of acute insult and to monitor the rhythm
   iv Chest radiograph: to check position of the endotracheal tube, and central line, to exclude a pneumothorax and other evidence of chest trauma, and signs of aspiration
   v Catheterize: to monitor urine output
   vi Specific therapy for hypotension, arrhythmias etc.

Chart of drugs and doses Table 6.

Reference

Evans, T. R. (ed.) (1990) *ABC of Resuscitation.* BMJ Publications, London

Case 31

A 48-year-old man presented with an 8-hour history of coarse tremor and sweating. He had been off work for the past 2 days with a cold. There was no history of thyroid disease, or other serious medical illness. He smoked, worked as a company director, and did not take any regular medication. His wife who accompanied him was extremely concerned about his condition.

On examination:

- Anxious
- Sweaty
- Apyrexial
- Pale

- Coarse tremor – most pronounced in the hands
- No goitre, thyroid bruit, or lid lag
- Pulse 100/min, blood pressure 160/100 mmHg
- No stigmata of chronic liver disease
- No liver flap
- Mental test score 10/10

Question

What is the diagnosis?

Answer

The primary diagnosis to consider in this man is alcohol withdrawal. The habitual drinker who abstains from alcohol is liable to develop symptoms of withdrawal. These take the form of a coarse tremor (morning shakes) associated with the signs of autonomic overactivity giving rise to sweating, flushing and a tachycardia. The condition has to be differentiated from thyrotoxicosis and acute anxiety states. Patient may deny a heavy alcohol intake even if specifically pressed on the subject.

This patient admitted to a heavy alcohol intake only after his wife had left. He mainly drank at work, concealing his addiction from his wife. Consequently, during the last 2 days, as he was at home with his wife, his alcohol consumption had dramatically decreased.

Alcohol withdrawal syndrome may progress, with the patient becoming increasingly anxious, restless and irritable. Convulsions may occur, and the patient becomes increasingly delirious.

The full blown syndrome of delirium tremens is characterized by a reduction in the level of conscious awareness, which usually manifests as acute disorientation. The patient has a poor attention span and memory, is vague and demonstrates pronounced fluctuation in mood. Perceptual disturbances including paranoia and hallucinations (the oft-quoted pink elephants!) occur. The associated physical symptoms and signs include ataxia, tremor, slurred speech and restlessness.

Korsakoff's (dysmnesic) syndrome should always be considered in these patients as many features of the two conditions are similar. In Korsakoff's syndrome the patient demonstrates an inability to retain any new information, and masks this by confabulating.

Management

i Consider alcohol withdrawal in any confused patient.
ii Oral chlormethiazole (4 capsules 4-hourly) or intravenous chlor-methiazole is the treatment of choice. The dose should be tailored to the

clinical response. Diazepam is an alternative. An initial oral dose of 20–30 mg, followed by 10 mg every 6 h for 48 h is very effective. This is nto recommended for outpatient treatment.

iii Give thiamine 100 mg i.v.

Outcome

This man was prescribed four capsules of chlormethiazole. Half an hour after taking them he had a generalized convulsion which had to be controlled with intravenous chlormethiazole.

Further notes

Alcohol is implicated as a contributing factor in a high proportion of injuries sustained at work. The CAGE questions are a very quick useful screening method of picking up high-risk problem drinkers.

The mnemonic CAGE stands for:

C: Have you tried to *cut down* your alcohol intake?
A: Do you drink *alone*?
G: Do you feel *guilty* about your alcohol intake?
E: Do you drink first thing in the morning (*eye opener*)?

Reference

Kennedy, H. J. (ed.) (1985) *Emergencies in Clinical Medicine.* Blackwell Scientific Publications, Oxford

Case 32

A man of 48 years was referred by his general practitioner to Accident and Emergency for an electrocardiogram. He had experienced chest pain intermittently for the past 48 h. The pain was a dull ache felt in the left upper chest, which was not associated with sweating or shortness of breath and did not radiate anywhere else. He had had four episodes of pain, each lasting about 1 h. Three episodes had occurred at night and had woken him from sleep, and one episode had occurred during his walk from the doctor's surgery to the hospital but he was now asymptomatic. There was no history of dyspepsia, exertional chest pain or a family history of ischaemic heart disease. He was a non-smoker and was not hypertensive. In the past month a consultant physician had organized a CT brain scan for chronic headaches. This scan was normal. There was no other relevant history.

110

On examination:

- Clinical examination was normal
- Blood pressure 140/85 mmHg, pulse 72/min regular
- Electrocardiogram normal

Questions

1 What is the most likely diagnosis?
2 What would you do if the man wanted to discharge himself claiming he had an important meeting to attend?

Answers

1 This man's pain should be considered ischaemic in nature until proven otherwise. The pain is somewhat atypical, and he has no risk factors, save being male and in the right age group. However, there is no other convincing diagnosis either from the history or examination. Therefore, he should be admitted and given intensive medical treatment as for unstable angina (see p. 182).

2 If the patient declines to stay, there is little you can do to stop him, but you should attempt to convince him of the errors of his action.

In the presence of a witness (senior nurse) you should explain the potential dangers of his action, including the potential of *death*. Any relatives should be advised of his condition and the possible consequences of his self-discharge. You should also ask a senior member of the Accident and Emergency staff to help you in this endeavour. If all this fails, he should be asked to sign a form which states that he is taking his own discharge against medical advice. You should clearly document in the patient's notes your advice, the presence of a witness and any other 'device' deployed to convince him to stay.

A completed self-discharge form in itself may not be sufficient to convince a court you tried hard enough to prevent this course of action.

If you consider that the patient has the 'capacity' to make these decisions concerning his own medical care there is nothing for you to do, save clearly documenting the interview.

One hour later this man returned to Accident and Emergency in an ambulance having 'fainted' during the meeting. He had chest pain, was sweaty and pale.

Clinical examination was again normal, although the monitor did reveal a self-limiting episode of atrial fibrillation.

A further electrocardiogram was performed which demonstrated an acute anterior infarction.

Whilst preparing to give the patient streptokinase he suddenly developed ventricular fibrillation.

Question

3 What is your management?

Answer

3 Ventricular fibrillation

Over 80% of patients sustaining a cardiac arrest will be found to be in ventricular fibrillation, and of the three arrhythmias commonly resulting in cardiac arrest (the other two being electromechanical dissociation and asystole) it has the best prognosis.

Treatment consists of DC cardioversion shock therapy. Defibrillation, that is, passing an electrical current through the heart, attempts to orchestrate the chaotic activity of the fibrillating myocardium by depolarizing a critical mass of it.

Current flow depends upon transthoracic impedance, and impedance can be reduced by ensuring:

i Correct positioning of the defibrillation paddles. The recommended positions are (a) one paddle to the right of the upper sternum, (b) one paddle to the left of the nipple in the mid axillary line.
ii Improving the contact between the electrode and skin by using electrode gel pads. *Note*: These should be replaced after being used for three shocks.
iii The electrode paddles are *firmly* applied to the chest wall.

Immediate management of ventricular fibrillation

a If you *witness* a cardiac arrest, or see ventricular fibrillation on the monitor, your first response should be a precordial thump. This is delivered by using the ulna border of the clenched fist brought down firmly into the lower third of the chest from a height of 20 cm.
b If unsuccessful and a defibrillator is close at hand, immediate defibrillation should be attempted three times with 200 joules, 200 joules and then 360 joules of energy before basic life support is commenced. In the absence of a defibrillator, basic life support (see Case 30) should be instituted. The resuscitation team called, and the defibrillator charged.
c The management of ventricular fibrillation should be in accordance with the guidelines suggested by the Resuscitation Council (UK).

Continue basic life support at all times
↓
Ventricular fibrillation
↓
Defibrillate 200 joules
↓
Defibrillate 200 joules
↓
Defibrillate 360 joules
↓
Adrenaline 1 mg i.v.
↓
Defibrillate 360 joules
↓
Lignocaine 100 mg i.v.
↓
Repeated defibrillations

If ventricular fibrillation is refractory to the above treatment consider:

i   repeat doses of adrenaline and lignocaine (total 3 mg/kg).
ii changing the paddle position of the defibrillator on the chest. For instance, one on the anterior chest and one placed below the tip of the left scapula.
iii change the defibrillator itself.
iv consider the use of other antidysrhythmic drugs such as bretylium tosylate 500 mg i.v. or amiodarone 300 mg i.v.
v   sodium bicarbonate should only be used when the arrest has been prolonged, that is greater than 15 min or to correct a documented acidosis.

(For a table of drugs used in cardiac arrest see p. 106.)

Outcome

Unfortunately this patient did not respond to the above therapy and after half an hour of active resuscitation he was pronounced dead.

Twenty minutes later the dead man's wife arrives in the Accident and Emergency department. Outline your approach to breaking bad news?

Answer

Breaking bad news

Breaking the news of a death to a relative is difficult. In the Accident and Emergency department the deaths that do occur are often unexpected and the result of a sudden illness or trauma. Some suggestions on how to deal with this difficult situation are found below.

General points

- Try not to appear distant, cold or rushed.
- These situations are highly emotional and it is not uncommon for you to experience some sad feelings.
- Do not ignore these emotions – empathy with the relatives will be appreciated.

Before you go in

- Take a moment to collect yourself mentally, and prepare yourself physically.
- Appear calm and neat, not dishevelled from the resuscitation room.
- Consider the most likely cause of death.
- Always go with an experienced nurse.

In the room

- Introduce yourself, and determine who is present and what their relationship to the deceased is. *This is very important.*
- Sit down and direct your remarks to the closest relation (wife, husband, daughter etc).
- Use simple language.
- Be truthful and direct, do not use euphemisms such as 'passed on' etc.
- Prepare them for the bad news with a statement such as, 'I'm sorry but I have some extremely bad news for you', then pause. Often they will suspect the worse, and will ask whether the person is dead. Having considered the possibility themselves often helps them to accept the situation more readily.
- You should repeat the news that the patient is dead.

On realizing the significance of the news there is generally a period of withdrawal. Reactions during this time can be varied, and sometimes very distressing. During this period of grief the relatives will not be able to accept any new information.

It is important to stay until this period of withdrawal is over, a return of eye contact and new questions will indicate the end of the retreat.

- Encourage them not to blame themselves.
- Allow them to see the body if desired.
- People with religious conviction may appreciate contact with an appropriate person e.g. rabbi, priest.
- A leaflet should be provided giving useful information about death certification and registration.
- Encourage relatives to return in the future if they feel the need to ask more questions.

Out of the room

- Inform the general practitioner.
- Look after yourself – take 5 min to reflect on the situation.

References

McCloughan, C. (1991) *Breaking bad news.* In *ABC of Major Trauma.* (eds P. Driscoll, D. Skinner and R. Earlham), BMJ Publications, London

Evans, T. R. (ed.) (1990) *ABC of Resuscitation.* BMJ Publications, London

Case 33

A woman presents with a 2-day history of an increasingly painful right eye. She complains of photophobia and blurred vision. There is no history of trauma or foreign body.

On examination:

- Visual acuity 6/12 right 6/6 left
- Red right eye, ciliary blush
- The pupil is miotic (small)

Question

What is the diagnosis?

Answer

The history is suggestive of anterior uveitis. Clinical examination should exclude an active keratitis as the two conditions give rise to similar symptoms.

Without the aid of a slit lamp it is easier to exclude an active keratitis than to confirm an active uveitis.

The following conditions giving rise to an acute keratitis should be considered:

- Foreign body or abrasion (see Case 2)
- Secondary to viral conjunctivitis
- Dendritic ulcer
- Marginal keratitis
- Corneal abscess

Herpes simplex infection can give rise to a conjunctivitis with or without an acute keratitis. The corneal lesion is typically a branching dendritic ulcer though it may start as a non-descript marginal corneal ulcer. Marginal keratitis may also be the result of an immune reaction, perhaps to the protein of a microorganism and rapidly resolves with steroid drops. However, it takes specialist knowledge to be able to differentiate between the two conditions, and there is no place for the administration of steroid drops by the Accident and Emergency staff.

Central corneal ulcers are usually bacterial in origin, and give rise to the symptoms of an acute keratitis with a marked loss of vision. Such ulcers are usually obvious and all need to be referred to the ophthalmology team.

Anterior uveitis

This condition gives rise to a painful red eye, and blurred vision. There is a distinct ciliary blush, and the pupil may be smaller than the normal side. Without the aid of a slit lamp, cells in the anterior chamber will not be seen, but a flare in the anterior chamber may be appreciated when a slit of light is passed obliquely into the anterior chamber.

Unlike keratitis there is usually less watering of the eye, and there is no foreign body sensation, otherwise symptoms are similar. All patients should be referred to the ophthalmology team.

Reference

Bron, A. J. and Davey, C. C. (1987) *The Unquiet Eye.* Glaxo Laboratories Ltd, Greenford

Case 34

A 24-year-old man arrives by ambulance. He had to be cut out of his car which he had driven into a brick wall at about 60 mph. The ambulance men inform you that the car was a 'write off', and that the front seat passenger was found dead in the car. They found the driver drowsy, complaining of chest and left hip pain. During the extrication they immobilized his neck in a rigid collar, provided oxygen and managed to establish a peripheral intravenous line through which had been run 500 ml of colloid. He arrived in the Accident and Emergency department awake and coherent. The trauma team and radiographers had been called.

The primary survey and resuscitation (see p. 167) revealed:

A	Airway	Talking, 60% oxygen mask in place
	Cervical spine	Immobilized in a rigid cervical collar

B	Breathing	Respiratory rate 24/min pink No clinical evidence of a pneumothorax, haemothorax, or flail segment

C	Circulation	No external haemorrhage
		Capillary return <2 s
		Cool peripheries
		Pulse 110/min irregular, blood pressure 90/70 mmHg
		Cardiac monitor sinus rhythm at 110 beats/min with
		    multiple ventricular ectopics
		A second peripheral line was established
		Blood taken for crossmatch of 6 units of blood, an
		    additional 1500 ml of colloid was given
		Arterial blood gases were taken

D	Disability	Glasgow coma score was 15 Both pupils were 4 mm, brisk light reflex Moved all fingers and toes
E	Exposure	Was complete, then he was covered with blankets

Radiographs of the chest, pelvis and lateral cervical spine were requested.

Secondary survey revealed the following:

Bruised forehead with a linear 3 cm laceration. Gentle digital exploration did not reveal an obvious skull fracture.

The patient claimed he had no neck symptoms.

No tenderness, crepitus, or swelling of the cervical spinous processes elicited.

Tramline bruising left by the seat belt extended across the right shoulder, down across the chest to the left anterior superior iliac spine of the pelvis.

Very tender and swollen midpoint of the manubrium sternum.

Abdomen – generalized tenderness, no guarding or rebound.

Bowel sounds present.

Rectal examination – normal sphincter tone, prostate normal, no blood.

No blood at urethral meatus.

Testes, scrotum and perineum normal.

No pain on springing the pelvis.

Tender around the left hip joint, left leg, internally rotated and flexed at the hip.

Bruising both knees.

Peripheral pulses present.

A nasogastric tube and a urinary catheter were inserted, and an electrocardiogram was performed.

Results

Radiographs

a	Chest (AP – supine film)	Mediastinum appeared widened No other obvious abnormality
b	Cervical spine (lateral view)	Normal
c	Pelvis	Pelvic ring intact Posterior dislocation of left hip Posterior lip of acetabulum fractured
d	Arterial blood gases on 60% oxygen	P_aO_2 13 kPa, P_aCO_2 4.2 kPa, pH 7.3, O_2 saturation 92%
e	Electrocardiogram	Tachycardia 114/min, multifocal ectopics Otherwise normal

At the end of the secondary survey:

f	Clinical observations	Respiratory rate 20/min, pulse 114 beats/min, blood pressure 100/70 mmHg Glasgow coma score 15

Questions

1 What is the importance of the mechanism of injury in this case?
2 What injuries do you suspect may be present?
3 What further history and examination is necessary in this patient?
4 What is your management?

Answers

1 Mechanism of injury

This man was involved in a high speed crash, resulting in a high energy deceleration type of injury. Speed is the most important predictor of the severity of injury in motor vehicle accidents. Often the actual speed of impact is unknown, but it can be inferred from the degree of damage to the vehicle. Other vital information indicating the severity of injury is the condition of the other occupants of the vehicle. Severe injuries, or fatalities among the other occupants suggest that serious injuries are to be expected in your patient, When a vehicle strikes a solid object, such as a brick wall, it comes to an abrupt halt. The occupants however, continue to travel at the initial speed until restrained by seat belts and/or the interior of the vehicle. For the driver, this is usually a combination of head and face against the windscreen, chest against the steering column, and knees against the dashboard, giving rise to a typical pattern of injuries. These are:

a *Mechanism: head and face against windscreen*
Head and facial injuries, contusions, fractures etc.
Neck injuries – transmitted to neck, as axial compression, flexion or extension injuries.

b *Mechanism: chest against steering wheel*

Chest wall injuries, e.g. rib fractures / flail segments — All possibly associated with a haemothorax or pneumothorax or both

Lung parenchyma, pulmonary laceration, or contusion

Cardiac contusion

Mediastinal injuries, rupture of a bronchus, rupture of the aorta

Thoracic spine injuries

Upper abdominal injury, ruptured diaphragm, liver/spleen

c *Mechanism: knee against the dashboard*
Knee injuries
Fractures to shaft or neck of femora
Dislocation of hip either central or posterior
Fractures of the pelvis

2 Suspected injuries

Injuries which should be suspected in this patient on completion of the secondary survey are:

a *Head injury*: contusion and laceration to the forehead. A skull radiograph is necessary to exclude a fracture.

b *Potential cervical spine injury*: the incidence of serious cervical spine injuries, in a conscious patient without neck symptoms, or localizing signs on examination is low. *However the neck should be completely immobilized until cervical radiographs are passed as normal by an experienced practitioner.*

c *Chest injuries*
   i *Clinical fracture of the sternum.*
   ii *Potential cardiac contusion*: contusion of the heart should always be suspected after a deceleration injury. The chest wall is brought to a halt by the steering wheel or seat belt, however the internal thoracic organs continue to move at the initial velocity giving rise to further injuries. Cardiac contusion is difficult to diagnose acutely. Patients complain of anterior chest pain, however, this is usually attributed to chest wall injury, in this case the fractured sternum.

The cardiac monitor and electrocardiogram may demonstrate multiple ventricular ectopics, atrial fibrillation, bundle branch block, or 'ST' changes. Alternatively, the only cardiac manifestation may be an unexplained tachycardia, which would be attributed to covert haemorrhage in the multiply-injured patient. With extensive damage cardiogenic shock may occur, this manifests as hypotension which is unresponsive to the administration of fluids. Serial electrocardiograms and enzymes are necessary, and cardiac imaging with ultrasound and radioisotopes may be helpful in making the diagnosis ultimately.

The cardiac monitor, demonstrated multiple ventricular ectopics in this man, which is suggestive of the diagnosis.

iii *Pulmonary contusion*: contusion to the lung is very common after serious blunt trauma to the chest. The incidence is greatest in patients with multiple rib fractures, and particularly flail segments. The chest X-ray may demonstrate diffuse alveolar shadowing, however this usually takes hours to develop. Such changes have to be differentiated from aspiration. Arterial blood gases are the most useful initial investigations. In the absence of other conditions which may compromise ventilation (e.g. flail segment, pneumothorax, hypotension), unexplained hypoxia should be taken as an indication of a pulmonary contusion.

In this man, on 60% oxygen a P_aO_2 of 13 kPa is abnormally low, and if breathing air he would certainly be severely hypoxic.

iv *Potential rupture of the aorta*: traumatic rupture of the aorta is the commonest cause of death after a deceleration injury. Tears in the aorta occur at the junction of the mobile arch, and the relatively fixed descending aorta at the ligamentum arteriosum. If complete rupture occurs as is usually the case, the patient dies at the scene.

If, however, the adventitial layer of the artery is left largely intact the patient may survive to reach hospital. In these patients blood slowly escapes into the mediastinum giving rise to a contained haematoma, and hypovolaemia. It is the haematoma which gives rise to the radiographic feature common to all cases of traumatic rupture, that of a widened mediastinum.

The mortality rate in these survivors is 50% for every day in hospital that the rupture is left untreated. A high index of suspicion is necessary. The finding of a widened mediastinum (>8 cm on a supine AP film) in a patient with a significant deceleration injury should always necessitate a cardiothoracic consultation. Other mediastinal injuries such as rupture of the bronchus, and diaphragmatic injuries are not suggested by the radiographic findings.

d *Potential abdominal injury*: the following points all suggest potential intra-abdominal injury:

i There is external evidence of injury, left by the tramline bruising of the seat belt.

ii The liver and spleen beneath the costal margins are vulnerable to injury from the steering wheel.

iii There is evidence of injury above and below the abdomen.

iv The abdomen is generally tender. (The presence or absence of bowel sounds being of no diagnostic significance.)

v After resuscitation with 2 l of fluid, the patient still has an unexplained tachycardia. There is no obvious source in the chest or pelvis to account for this.

All the above points would be an indication for further investigation. Peritoneal lavage is the investigation of choice. (See Further notes.)

e *Posterior dislocation of the left hip.*

f *Contusion to the left knee.*

3 Further history and examination

Essential further history includes:

a Further details of the accident if available from the patient. Were alcohol and/or drugs involved?

b Serious past medical history: all significant details should be documented.

c Previous or current medications including steroids and allergies.

d Details of the time they last ate and drank. Important from the anaesthetic point of view as is the history of previous anaesthetic problems.

e Tetanus status.

f Next of kin – contact number.

It is important to obtain this information early as clinical deterioration may prevent it being obtained later.

Further examination

It is important that the head-to-toe examination is very thorough. Missing a wrist fracture, or a knee haemarthrosis could have serious long-term consequences for the patient.

All trauma patients should be log rolled onto their side so that a thorough examination of the whole spine, renal, area and buttocks may take place. Such a manoeuvre should be delayed until the lateral cervical spine film has been passed as normal.

4 Management

Continued management consists of:

a Continuous oxygen 60% via Venturi mask.

b After 2 l fluid replacement, blood is necessary. The sustained tachycardia indicates the possibility of continued bleeding.

c Peritoneal lavage should be performed. Active bleeding in the abdomen has to be excluded. A positive result would indicate the need for a laparotomy.

d The hip needs relocating.

e An aortogram is necessary to exclude a rupture of the aorta. The cardiothoracic surgeons should be contacted.

f The scalp, and knee wounds need to be sutured and dressed. Tetanus should be administered if required.

g Full documentation of the history, examination, investigations and treatment given is necessary.

Outcome

Peritoneal lavage was performed on this patient. On insertion of the catheter, 20 ml of frank blood were aspirated. The patient was taken to theatre, and at laparotomy the spleen was removed. During the same anaesthetic the left hip was relocated. A brachial artery catheter was inserted and an aortogram was performed. This was normal.

He was transferred to the Intensive Care Unit where he was electively ventilated overnight due to poor oxygen saturations. He was extubated the next day.

Serial electrocardiograms and enzymes were normal. He spent 3 weeks in hospital, and was then allowed home. He was reviewed in the orthopaedic outpatient clinic.

Further notes

Indications for peritoneal lavage in the multiple injured patient

The diagnosis of intra-abdominal injury after trauma can be very difficult. This is due to:

1 As many as 20% of patients with significant intra-abdominal injuries have no clinical signs at presentation.

2 Patients with injuries to the lower chest, pelvis and back can make the interpretation of the physical signs difficult.

3 Patients with altered consciousness, cord lesions, or who are drunk or drugged may have absent/altered signs.

Diagnostic peritoneal lavage is 98% sensitive for intraperitoneal bleeding and has superseded other diagnostic methods such as the four quadrant tap. It is, however, an operative procedure and should be performed by the surgical team under whose care the patient is admitted, (or in their presence).

Indications for peritoneal lavage are:

- Equivocal abdominal signs
- History of significant blunt thoracoabdominal trauma
- Unexplained tachycardia, or hypotension
- Associated lower chest or pelvic injuries
- If the patient will be transferred to another specialist unit (e.g. neurosurgical) and there is any doubt about the significance of the abdominal examination
- If the patient will be unavailable for monitoring, e.g. prolonged orthopaedic operation.

Contra-indications:

- Relative
  Previous abdominal operations
  Morbid obesity
  Coagulopathy
  Advanced cirrhosis
- Patients with advanced pregnancy, or pelvic fractures, should be lavaged through an incision above the umbilicus.

Reference

Driscoll, P., Skinner, D. and Earlham, R. (eds) (1991) *ABC of Major Trauma*. BMJ Publications, London

Case 35

A 38-year-old woman presented with a 6-h history of pain in the left upper quadrant of her abdomen, associated with an ache in her left shoulder. She woke with the pain, which was exacerbated by inspiration and by lying down. Lying down made her so uncomfortable that she was very reluctant to do so. Two months previously she had her appendix removed, and had made an uncomplicated recovery. She had been well up until that day without any history of respiratory or renal illness. Her bowel habit had been normal. She had missed her last period 3 weeks previously and she had put this down to having had the operation. Her periods had been otherwise completely regular, and she denied any irregular bleeding, or lower abdominal pain. She had been using the cap. There was no other significant past medical history.

On examination:

- Well, apyrexial
- Pulse 98/min, blood pressure 125/70 mmHg
- Chest clear, no rubs
- Abdomen tender left upper and lower quadrants
- No guarding, or rebound tenderness
- Bowel sounds normal
- Rectal examination normal
- Urine clear

Questions

1 What is your initial diagnosis?
2 What is your management?

Answers

1 The initial working diagnosis should be of free intraperitoneal blood. The pain has the features of diaphragmatic irritation. These are that the pain is exacerbated by inspiration, lying down, and radiates to the shoulder. In a young woman the most likely diagnosis is a ruptured ectopic pregnancy. Other potential causes should be considered once this condition has been excluded.

2 Initial management should be:

- Establish venous access
- Take blood for crossmatch of 4 units
- Commence fluid infusion 500 ml (colloid, crystalloid)
- Urgent pregnancy test

Note: the routine pregnancy slide tests available in Accident and Emergency department, are relatively cheap (e.g. Clear View) and are quick to perform. However, they are not very sensitive, with an appreciable false-negative rate. The incidence of false positives is however low, and therefore a positive result can be relied upon. However a more sensitive test (e.g. urinary or serum beta-HCG) is necessary when it is essential to exclude early pregnancy, when the slide test is negative.

In patients in whom you are convinced that the diagnosis is an ectopic pregnancy the pelvic examination should be deferred and the gynaecology team contacted immediately.

In patients in whom there is clinical uncertainty, having established venous access, pelvic examination is necessary. Evidence of cervical excitation, adnexal masses and tenderness should be specifically sought.

In this woman the pelvic examination was normal, and urinary beta-HCG was negative, making an ectopic pregnancy highly unlikely. An alternative gynaecological pathology that may rarely give rise to this presentation would be an ovarian catastrophe (rupture of a cyst, torsion). A normal pelvic examination again would assist in excluding this diagnosis.

What alternative diagnoses should you consider now?

1 Basal pneumonia

A clinically silent basal pneumonic process or viral pleurisy could be responsible and a chest radiograph is necessary.

2 Subphrenic collection

The recent appendicectomy may well predispose this woman to such a collection, however the history is unusually short, and patients generally appear quite unwell in the presence of chronic sepsis. A chest radiograph revealing a raised hemidiaphragm or sympathetic pleural effusion would be suggestive, and a full blood count might demonstrate a leucocytosis.

3 Pancreatitis

It would be uncommon for pancreatitis to present in this way. However as the pain is more likely to be due to an atypical presentation of a common condition, rather than to an uncommon one, the amylase should be estimated.

In this woman the chest radiograph was normal and the white cell count was 5.3. Amylase was 120 iu.

Question

What would your management be now?

Answer

Further investigation is clearly necessary, and without any obvious diagnosis the patient needs to be referred to the surgeons for admission and further evaluation. Abdominal ultrasound examination would be the next investigation of choice.

Uncommon cases of free intraperitoneal fluid

Uncommon conditions which can give rise to free intraperitoneal blood include spontaneous rupture of the spleen, and the rare condition of splenic artery aneurysm.

Spontaneous rupture of the spleen may occur in the months following a viral illness such as glandular fever. Normal spleens do not spontaneously rupture.

Cautionary tale
A male aged 27 presented with severe left upper quadrant and shoulder tip pain, pallor and a tachycardia. He was a heavy drinker, and gave a history of glandular fever 6 months previously. The initial diagnosis was acute on chronic pancreatitis although his amylase was only 213 iu. Ultrasound examination 24 h after admission revealed a large splenic haematoma with free intraperitoneal fluid.

The condition of splenic artery aneurysm is very rare, and normally occurs in young and middle-aged females. The aneurysms have a propensity to bleed particularly during pregnancy.

It is mentioned here solely because the ultrasound examination performed on this woman demonstrated a large aneurysm of the splenic artery and some free intraperitoneal fluid. A surprise to all concerned.

Outcome

The patient underwent a splenectomy, and made an uneventful recovery.

Reference

London, J. D. O. Chapter 42 in *Hamilton Bailey's Emergency Surgery*, 11th edn. Wright, Bristol, 445

Case 36

A 3-year-old child is brought to the Accident and Emergency department by her parents. She is crying and not using her left arm. On further questioning it transpires that the family are on holiday in London, and when travelling by underground the child refused to enter the carriage. Realizing that she was either going to be trapped in the doors, or left on the platform, her father pulled her briskly on-board. The parents both date her distress to this incident. The child herself is unable to give any useful information.

Questions

1 What is the likely diagnosis?
2 Is investigation appropriate?
3 What is the management?
4 What advice should be given to the parents?

Answers

1 Pulled elbow. The history, which is typically a sudden jerk on the extended elbow, is characteristic of a pulled elbow. In young children, under the age of 4–6 years, the head of the radius is cylindrical rather than conical and can easily sublux through the annular ligament. As the child grows, normal development of the radial head makes the injury less likely to occur.

2 Radiological investigation is unnecessary, where the history is highly suggestive of a pulled elbow. If performed the radiograph is likely to be entirely normal and subluxation of the radial head will not be evident. If there is clinical suspicion of a more serious injury to the elbow, the radiograph should be carried out in the normal way, taking a view of the uninjured side if radiological advice is not immediately available.

3 A subluxed radial head is reduced by fully supinating the elbow, which is flexed to 90°. Gentle pressure exerted towards the elbow generally results in a palpable and occasionally an audible click over the radial head. Usually the child will start to use the arm normally within 30 min. The parents should be asked to return the following day if movement in the arm has not returned to normal.

4 This minor injury is often recurrent. Parents should be advised to avoid swinging children by their hands, and to grasp the upper arm if lifting or pulling the child. They should also be shown the method of reducing the subluxation if the history is highly suggestive of this injury. They should however be told to bring the child to the Accident and Emergency department if two attempts fail.

Case 37

A 72-year-old man was brought to the Accident and Emergency department acutely short of breath. No history was available from the man himself as he was too breathless to speak, but his wife accompanied him and was able to provide the following information. Over the past 10 years he has suffered with a 'bad chest' and was 'under the hospital'. He had been admitted four times in the last 2 years with bronchitis. Any cold appeared 'to go to his chest'. He had been taking the following medication: salbutamol and steroid inhalers, aminophylline and a diuretic since his last admission 8 months ago. He was normally able to walk 15–20 yards (13.7–18.2 m) on the flat without getting short of breath.

During the last 36 h, however, he had become progressively shorter of breath at rest and had experienced some aching left-sided chest pain. He had had paroxysms of coughing, but failed to produce any sputum. She felt that this episode was very similar to the previous illness which resulted in hospitalization.

She was not aware that he had ever had any heart trouble or hypertension, although there was a history of peptic ulceration treated surgically 20 years ago. There was no history of asthma and he smoked five cigarettes a day.

On examination:

- Acutely short of breath
- Unable to speak
- Cyanosed
- Apyrexial
- Respiratory rate of 28/min
- Using accessory muscles of respiration
- Barrel-shaped chest
- Trachea central
- Widespread wheezes bilaterally
- No crepitations
- Pulse 112/min, blood pressure 160/105 mmHg
- Cool peripheries with small volume pulse
- JVP elevated 2 cm
- Heart sounds difficult to hear, but no obvious added sounds
- Abdomen soft, smooth enlarged liver
- Bilateral ankle oedema

Questions

1 What is your working diagnosis?
2 What is your immediate management?

Answers

1 The working diagnosis is an acute exacerbation of chronic airflow limitation, but asthma should always be considered.

The history of a chronic chest problem, with repeated hospital admissions and poor exercise tolerance all point to chronic airflow limitation. Most commonly this is an irreversible condition of the airways, and is the result of chronic heavy smoking. Reversible airway disease (asthma) would be strongly suggested if this patient had never smoked, or had a history of asthma (chronic cough, poor exercise tolerance) as a child.

Infection is the commonest cause of an acute exacerbation of chronic airflow limitation, though other precipitating causes should be always considered and actively excluded.

These include:

- Pneumonia: either picked up clinically, because of the signs of consolidation, or evidenced by new shadowing of the chest radiograph.

- Pneumothorax: a pneumothorax can be fatal in a patient with airflow limitation and the initial examination should always attempt positively to exclude this diagnosis. A small pneumothorax can be difficult to detect clinically and a chest radiograph is necessary. Remember that a pneumothorax needs to be differentiated from an emphysematous bulla.

- Pulmonary oedema: co-existing pulmonary oedema may be very difficult to exclude clinically, as basal crepitations may be absent, wheezes being the only auscultatory evidence of raised pulmonary venous pressure. Equally other clinical signs such as a raised jugular venous pressure or triple rhythm can be difficult to detect in the acutely breathless patient with a very noisy chest. A chest radiograph again is a very useful indicator of raised pulmonary venous pressure. Care should be exercised when interpreting the radiographic signs in a patient with a hyperinflated chest as signs of pulmonary oedema can be quite subtle (cardiomegaly and upper lobe blood diversion, may be less obvious). An electrocardiogram will be necessary to exclude an acute ischaemic event.

- Pulmonary embolus: sudden onset of shortness of breath associated with chest pain should always raise the possibility of embolus. Further evidence from the clinical history, electrocardiogram, chest radiograph and arterial blood gases should be sought. However, the diagnosis can be very difficult to make clinically, and ventilation perfusion scanning is often necessary, though the results in patients with chronic airflow limitation are often impossible to interpret.

2 Immediate management consists of:

- Strong verbal reassurance
- 24% oxygen via a Venturi mask
- Nebulized salbutamol 5 mg with the addition of 500 µg of ipratropium bromide.
- And the following urgent investigations:
  a chest radiograph: to exclude the conditions listed above. Specific

therapy will be necessary depending upon the findings. In particular, a diuretic for pulmonary oedema, and drainage of a pneumothorax.

b Arterial blood gases: the degree of hypoxia, hypercapnia, and acidosis needs to be documented early. Therapeutic options will depend upon the results (see below).

c electrocardiogram: evidence of ischaemia, or changes compatible with pulmonary embolus should be sought.

Additional therapy

In the absence of an obvious precipitating cause for this deterioration, additional therapy consists of:

- Controlled oxygen therapy (see below)
- Salbutamol and ipatropium nebulizers 6-hourly
- Hydrocortisone 200 mg i.v. stat then 100 mg 8-hourly or prednisolone 30 mg p.o. if tolerated
- Intravenous ampicillin 1 g 6-hourly for infection (+ erythromycin 500 mg 6-hourly for new chest radiograph shadowing)
- The use of aminophylline is controversial. Many authorities believe that a loading dose is too dangerous to give to a severely hypoxic patient because of the potential serious side effects (even if the patient has not been on the drug at home). A maintenance dose of 250 mg over 8 h (0.5 mg/kg/h) as a continuous infusion is associated with a lower incidence of side effects and is usually more acceptable.

  You should be guided by the department's policy regarding this matter
- Diuretics for associated right heart failure as evidence by a raised jugular venous pressure, hepatomegaly, and peripheral oedema, are not of immediate benefit or importance. Indeed peripheral oedema in the absence of other features of heart failure may well respond to oxygen therapy, without the need for diuretics.
- Physiotherapy – forced expiratory technique.

The medical team should be called to admit the patient.

Outcome

The chest radiograph demonstrated hyperinflated lungs without evidence of infection, pneumothorax or pulmonary oedema, and the electrocardiogram revealed changes compatible with anterior ischaemia.

Arterial blood gases revealed a P_aO_2 5.7 kPa, P_aCO_2 6.3 kPa, pH 7.22, bicarbonate 32, O_2 sat 72% (on 24% oxygen). He was then given 28% oxygen. Repeat blood gases demonstrated a P_aO_2 6.5 kPa, P_aCO_2 7.8 kPa and a pH of 7.18.

Consequently he was treated with doxapram and continuous 28% oxygen therapy, diuretics, steroids, antibiotics, and bronchodilators. Six hours after admission, the situation had not significantly improved, and the patient was exhausted. He was therefore ventilated. Despite intensive therapy he died while being ventilated 4 days later.

Further notes

1 Respiratory failure

Respiratory failure occurs when the lungs are unable to maintain normal gas exchange at rest, and is arbitrarily defined as finding a P_aO_2 of below 8 kPa, ($SaO_2 < 90$) or a P_aCO_2 above 6.7 kPa. Hypoxaemic respiratory failure (type 1) is said to occur when the $P_aO_2 < 8$ kPa, but the P_aCO_2 is normal or low. This is due to ventilation/perfusion mismatching and occurs in conditions such as asthma, pneumonia and pulmonary oedema. In ventilatory failure (type 2) there is alveolar hypoventilation which leads to retention of CO_2 with or without hypoxia. The commonest cause of this type of respiratory failure is chronic airflow limitation. Other causes include depression of the respiratory centre with sedative drugs and opiates, acute brain insults (such as head injury or cerebral haemorrhage), deranged chest wall mechanics (e.g. flail chest) or neuromuscular diseases.

In patients with irreversible chronic airflow limitation there is an element of both hypoxaemic and ventilatory failure giving rise to hypoxaemia and hypercapnia.

Clinically the signs of respiratory failure can be overlooked, and there is no substitute for performing arterial blood gases estimations. Central cyanosis is the cardinal sign of hypoxia and is most easily seen in the lips or tongue when viewed in a good light. Hypercapnia gives rise to vasodilatation with warm hands, bounding pulses, headache, drowsiness and rarely papilloedema.

Tissue oxygen delivery depends upon the haemoglobin concentration (g/dl), oxygen saturation (%), and the cardiac output. Whereas there is little change in oxygen saturation when the P_aO_2 drops down to 8 kPa below this level there is a large fall in oxygen saturation with further falls in the P_aO_2. When the P_aO_2 falls below 6 kPa it is life threatening. Therefore treatment aims to increase oxygen delivery to the tissues by treating shock and thereby improving perfusion, and by judicious oxygen therapy to raise the P_aO_2 to above 8 kPa. In some patients with severe chronic airflow limitation, this may be impossible as their 'normal' P_aO_2 when well may be below 8 kPa. In these patients values over 7 kPa are acceptable.

2 Oxygen therapy

In patients in type 1 respiratory failure correction of the hypoxaemia is attempted by increasing the inspired oxygen concentration using a 60% Venturi mask. Lack of respiratory drive is not a problem in these patients, and there is little danger of allowing CO_2 retention.

If the hypoxaemia fails to correct by increasing oxygen concentrations, ventilation should be considered.

In patients with type 2 failure, treatment of the underlying causes is necessary (i.e. reverse opioid overdose with naloxone), but if this is not possible immediately as with an acute head injury, elective ventilation will be necessary.

Patients with chronic obstructive airways disease with both hypoxaemia and hypercapnia may need controlled oxygen therapy. The aim in these patients is to correct the life-threatening hypoxia by attempting to raise the $P_{O_2} > 8$ kPa. However, in doing so the P_aCO_2 may rise, as the oxygen diminishes their respiratory drive. The reason for this hypoventilation in patients with chronic hypercapnia is thought to be due to the fact that the respiratory centre is no longer sensitive to small changes in the P_aCO_2, hypoxaemia being the main respiratory stimulus. If the hypoxia is quickly reversed, the patient hypoventilates allowing CO_2 accumulation.

The aim in these patients therefore is to correct hypoxia without allowing significant CO_2 retention. This can be difficult to achieve.

Initially these patients should be given 24% oxygen by Venturi mask. The arterial blood gases should be measured regularly, and the inspired oxygen concentration should be varied to find the F_1O_2 which best corrects the hypoxia without provoking a rise in the $P_{CO_2} > 7$ kPa (or by 1.5 kPa).

If the hypoxia is impossible to improve by these means then respiratory stimulants, or ventilation should be considered.

Reference

Davis, R. J. Chapter 12 in *Clinical Medicine*. (eds Kumar and Clark) (1st edn 1987). Baillière Tindall, Eastbourne, 551

Case 38

A 29-year-old woman is brought to the Accident and Emergency department in the early hours of the morning, by the police. She is weeping and distressed and gives the history that while making her way home from a party she was the victim of a vicious assault and was raped. She denies loss of consciousness but says that she was hit about the face and head, and kicked in the chest, abdomen and loin.

Questions

1 Outline your management of this patient.
2 Who should carry out the pelvic examination?
3 What are your responsibilities to this patient?

Answers

1 The initial assessment of this patient involves taking a full history to ascertain what injuries might have occurred and then to carry out a full physical examination to exclude serious head, chest or abdominal injuries. Provided there is no evidence of heavy vaginal bleeding indicating a potentially serious perineal or vaginal injury, the rape aspect may be temporarily put to one side while other injuries are assessed and appropriately investigated. Once the patient's head, chest and abdominal injuries have been assessed, and any necessary treatment instituted, the patient may be referred onto the police surgeon. This may be either in the Accident and Emergency department or preferably in a designated suite at the police station (known as a victim examination suite) where the police surgeon may see and examine the patient.

Obviously, patients who have been the victims of a violent assault are very distressed and require a particularly sensitive approach with careful explanations of the examination and findings. It is important that even at a very early stage in the patient's assessment that a non-judgemental approach is adopted whether or not the casualty officer believes the background history. The police have now adopted a policy of investigating rape in a much more active manner and it has been shown that the patient's ability to get over such an attack often depends on the initial attitudes displayed and any suggestion to the patient that they may have put themselves at risk of such an attack are not likely to be helpful.

It is vital that no evidence of possible forensic value is lost. If the patient is undressed in the Accident and Emergency department, as is clearly necessary for a full examination, this should be performed over a sheet of brown paper, and her clothes assembled over a similar sheet so that any hairs or fibres from her skin or clothing may be retained for forensic examination. All her clothing must be retained and, if it has been removed it should be placed in bags which should be signed by the person responsible so that a chain of evidence may be maintained. The patient should not wash or bathe until the forensic examination is complete. The forensic examination should not be delayed other than through clinical necessity as the more rapidly it is carried out, the more evidence may be gathered.

2 Ideally a police surgeon should carry out a pelvic examination so that a full forensic evaluation may be undertaken. Sometimes, for a variety of reasons, a woman may refuse to involve the police following an assault, including rape. Although it is preferable for the police to be involved in such a serious assault and gentle efforts of persuasion are appropriate, to inform the police against the patient's wishes would constitute a serious breach of confidentiality.

Under these circumstances a full examination, including a pelvic examination, may be carried out either in the Accident and Emergency department or in the department of Genitourinary Medicine.

Women may request a female doctor to see and examine them and, if at all possible, their wishes should be complied with. At night, when there may not be genitourinary medicine cover available on site, the on-call registrar in gynaecology will probably be the most appropriate doctor. Few casualty officers, unless they are experienced in gynaecology or genitourinary medicine will have had the breadth of experience required to undertake the examination and initial counselling.

A few Accident and Emergency departments now have the facilities and expertise to carry out an appropriate forensic examination so that if a patient later changes her mind about involving the police, the forensic evidence has already been taken and is available. However, this is not universal and the patient should be warned that, in general, forensic evidence will not be collected and if there is any possibility that she might wish to press charges, it is vital that a police surgeon is involved from the outset.

3 The casualty officer dealing with a patient who has been raped has the following responsibilities:

a To look for other serious or potentially life-threatening injuries, to treat them appropriately and record them carefully and accurately in the notes. All bruising, scratch marks, bite marks, abrasions and lacerations should be carefully noted and their measured size recorded.

b The patient should be made aware of the possibility of contracting a sexually transmitted disease as a result of the assault. If the patient refuses to involve the police then a forensic examination will not be carried out, except in certain Accident and Emergency departments which have undertaken to do this. It is therefore not necessary to perform a formal pelvic examination to take swabs unless there is evidence that the patient has a pre-existing sexually transmitted disease. Perineal injuries should be carefully recorded but it may not be appropriate to perform a pelvic examination at the initial visit.

If the patient presents to the Accident and Emergency department some time after the rape has taken place then investigations for sexually transmitted disease should be carried out.

The following investigations are appropriate:

i take serum for hepatitis serology (save serum HIV status), and syphilis serology.

ii high vaginal swab (into Stuart's transport medium) for *Trichomonas vaginalis*, candida or bacterial vaginosis.

iii endocervical swabs for gonorrhoea and chlamydia (two separate swabs, one in charcoal transport medium and one in chlamydia culture medium).

iv rectal and oral swabs should be taken in the same way.

The patient should be asked to attend the department of Genitourinary Medicine for examination at approximately 10 days from the time of the rape. Seeing the patient sooner may be appropriate to initiate counselling but given the incubation period for sexually transmitted diseases, there is no need to take pelvic swabs earlier than this other than for forensic reasons. If the patient presents to the Accident and Emergency department some time after she has been raped with symptoms suggestive of a sexually transmitted disease, swabs should be taken, she should be treated with an appropriate antibiotic and referred onto the department of Genitourinary Medicine for further counselling and test of cure.

The use of prophylactic antibiotics to prevent sexually transmitted disease in rape is not advised except in very exceptional circumstances such as when an intrauterine contraceptive has been fitted. Should the patient feel that she has been raped by a person who is likely to transmit hepatitis B then it may be appropriate to give an accelerated course of vaccine unless the perpetrator is available for hepatitis serology to be analysed, in which case it may be appropriate to give the immunoglobulin if a patient is proven positive.

c To cover the possibility of pregnancy resulting from this attack, should the woman not be on the oral contraceptive pill, arrangements must be made for her to have the morning after pill if she is within child-bearing age. Ovran (levonorgestrel 250 µg and ethinyloestradiol 50 mg) two tablets taken within 72 h and a further two tablets after 12 h should be prescribed. The patient should be reviewed within 3 weeks to ensure compliance and to inquire whether vomiting followed the administration of this medication.

If the patient presents after 72 h but before 5 days then consideration should be given to fitting an intrauterine contraceptive device. This would clearly be done in conjunction with either the department of Genitourinary Medicine or the gynaecologists and should be covered with the administration of doxycycline 100 mg b.d. for a week.

d Counselling. Vicious personal assault, particularly rape, is an intensely distressing and damaging event and adequate counselling is vital. The evidence suggests that the earlier the counselling is instituted, the better the outlook for the patient. Counselling may be arranged through the police or through the department of Genitourinary Medicine. Alternatively the Victim Support Group offers a 24-h national service where the patient can be accompanied by a volunteer to the police station and subsequently to the department of Genitourinary Medicine and contact may be maintained for up to a year.

This service not only covers female rape but male rape and physical assault. An alternative counselling agency is Rape Crisis.

Case 39

A 7-week-old boy was brought to the Accident and Emergency department by his parents. They were concerned because the child had been vomiting after every feed for the last 3 days. The vomiting had on occasions been projectile in that it would land 2–3 feet away but in the main consisted of possetting. (That is, simple regurgitation which ended up on the child's clothes or the parents shoulders!) The child had been eager to feed initially despite the vomiting, but over the last 18 h he had lost interest and was rather listless and feverish. The vomit did not contain any blood or bile and there had not been any diarrhoea.

The child had been born by vaginal delivery at term, after an uneventful pregnancy and weighed 3.4 kg. He had been bottle fed since birth on Cow & Gate Premium and usually took between 7–8 oz (200–225 ml) five times a day. In the clinic one week prior to the illness he weighed 4.35 kg.

The parents had two other children aged 2 and 4.5 years, who were both well.

On examination:

- Apyrexial
- Weight 4.23 kg
- The child looked pale, and was quiet
- Dry mucous membranes
- Fontanelle was normal
- Skin turgor was normal
- Ears and throat not inflamed
- Respiratory rate 30/min, pulse 130/min
- Abdomen soft with no palpable masses
- Bowel sounds were normal
- No nappy rash, and no herniae

Questions

1 What is the differential diagnosis?
2 What would be your management of this child?

Answers

1 Differential diagnosis

The differential diagnosis should include:

- Pyloric stenosis
- Urinary tract infection
- Intercurrent viral infection
- Gastro-oesophageal reflux
- Feeding problems

Pyloric stenosis

Pyloric stenosis occurs in 3 babies per 1000, between the ages of 2 and 12 weeks, and is much more common in boys (M:F; 4:1). The typical picture is of the active, hungry male infant who has projectile vomiting after feeds. If visible peristalsis and a palpable tumour are found after a test feed then the diagnosis is not in doubt.

Many infants, however, present with evidence of dehydration and weight loss on a background of vomiting and the child appears apathetic. Weight loss and electrolyte disturbance are common, as is constipation.

The diagnosis is made by observing visible peristalsis or finding a pyloric 'tumour' after a test feed. Ultrasound or barium meal examination may be necessary if this is absent.

Definitive treatment is rehydration and surgery.

Urinary tract infection/intercurrent viral infections

This clinical picture also occurs with infections, particularly urinary tract infection and otitis media, but other infections such as pneumonia or meningitis should be borne in mind.

In infants less than 2 months old urinary tract infection is commoner in males, and can present in a variety of non-specific ways such as lethargy and poor feeding, vomiting, poor weight gain, intermittent pyrexia, irritability and excessive crying. As a consequence a clean catch urine sample should be examined in all infants who are non-specifically unwell. At this age there is a high incidence of both structural and functional abnormalities (posterior urethral valves and ureteric reflux) leading to incomplete bladder emptying. There is a high risk of renal scarring if this goes undetected.

Gastro-oesophageal reflux

Many children have innocent regurgitation of feeds, because the functional lower oesophageal sphincter is not well established in early infancy. However, this is not a problem if the child is otherwise well, thriving, and gaining weight satisfactorily. The infant's weight should always be checked on a centile chart.

Reflux can occasionally, particularly when associated with a hiatus hernia, give rise to constitutional upset in the infant. There can be large volume vomits, which may be blood streaked. These babies may be very irritable while feeding and fail to thrive, and should be assessed by the paediatricians.

Treatment initially consists of thickening the feeds with carob preparations or cornflour and sitting the child up. Antacids may also be helpful.

Feeding problem

Vomiting can be the presenting symptom in infants who are overfed. On average an infant's daily milk intake should be about 150 ml/kg, and values grossly in excess of this may be responsible for vomiting. (This baby was being given over 250 ml/kg).

Infants who are being continually disturbed at feeding times due to the lack of a quiet, calm environment, over anxious parents or problems with milk supply due to defective teats, may also have persistent vomiting. Vomiting in these instances is usually present from soon after birth and is brought to light by a period of observation on the ward.

However, the history given by this baby's parents suggests an acute illness rather than a feeding problem.

2 Management

This child needs to be referred to the paediatrician on call for admission when the following can be arranged:

- Urea and electrolytes should be taken to exclude a hypokalaemic, hypochloraemic alkalosis which might complicate pyloric stenosis.
- A sterile urine sample should be collected to exclude a urinary tract infection.
- A test feed should be performed, and visible peristalsis and a palpable pylorus (pyloric tumour) sought.

Outcome

This boy had pyloric stenosis. He was rehydrated over a period of 24 h, and then taken to theatre. Following a Ramstedt procedure, milk feeding was reintroduced and the boy made a quick and uneventful recovery.

Reference

Baur, L. A. and Walker-Smith, J. A. (1989) Infant feeding problems. *Update*, 1 November, 799

Case 40

A 45-year-old man presents with a 3-day history of a discharging right ear. The discharge is green and smelly and has persisted despite a course of antibiotics prescribed by his general practitioner. He also complains that he appears to be more deaf in that ear than normal. In the past he recalled a similar episode 5 years previously which got better quickly on ear drops, but he felt he had been slightly deaf in that ear ever since. He had not had any surgery on his ears or other significant past medical history.

On examination:

- There was mucopus in the external auditory meatus which precluded visualizing the canal or drum
- Pressure on the tragus was not uncomfortable, and it did not precipitate vertigo
- Rinne's test was negative

Questions

1 What is the diagnosis?
2 What is the significance of Rinne's test?
3 What is the management?

Answers

1 Two conditions commonly give rise to discharging ear, namely otitis externa and chronic otitis media. (Acute otitis media normally presents with pain rather than discharge.) The history can be very helpful to help to differentiate between the two.

Otitis externa

Otitis externa is common, and although it may present with pain it usually presents with an irritating, itchy ear, which discharges pus. The associated hearing loss is typically minimal. A combination of factors predispose to this condition including: trauma (from cotton buds etc.), a hot, damp environment, and local skin diseases, e.g. eczema. Pressure on the tragus is often uncomfortable, and the canal appears red, swollen and congested. The drum if seen should be intact.

Chronic otitis media

In chronic otitis media, discharge (mucopus) is the rule rather than pain as the chronic perforation of the drum does not allow the pressure to build up. In some patients the perforation predisposes to repetitive infection, whereas others have long asymptomatic periods. Some hearing impairment is usually noticed by the patient, which is more pronounced than that associated with otitis externa, and there is no associated itchiness of the ear. Examination may reveal a perforation of the drum, or evidence of disease in the attic (cholesteatomas).

A history of vertigo is ominous. This symptom should always be enquired about in a patient with a discharging ear, as chronic middle ear infection may predispose to a fistula of the semicircular canal. If pressure on the tragus produces vertigo then this is suggestive of a fistula (a positive fistula sign). A fistula may allow contiguous spread of infection from the middle ear or intracranially.

2 A Rinne's negative test suggests that there is a conductive cause for the deafness as bone conduction is better than air conduction (Rinne's negative when hearing loss >20 dB). This reversal of the normal situation may favour chronic otitis media rather than otitis externa, as a cause for the discharging ear.

Chronic otitis media may be associated with either a large perforation, or ossicular disruption and both may give rise to a significant conductive loss.

The Rinne's tuning fork test is performed using a 512 Hz fork which is activated and held by the external canal, and then placed on the mastoid process behind the same ear. The patient is asked in which position the fork is heard the loudest. Normally it is loudest when the fork is held by the external auditory meatus. This is called Rinne's positive, that is air conduction is better than bone conduction.

If the patient cannot decide in which position the fork is heard the loudest then the test is repeated. This time the fork is held by the external meatus until the sound is no longer heard, and then placed on the mastoid process. If the patient then hears it here this is a negative result (i.e. bone conduction is better than air conduction).

3 The initial management in this patient is the same irrespective of the underlying diagnosis. A swab should be taken for culture and sensitivity. Good aural toilet is essential to aid recovery in both conditions and allow auroscopic examination of the canal and drum. Ideally this should be performed with an operating microscope, however, a piece of cotton wool on an orange stick is usually sufficient and much more readily available. Effective aural toilet should allow inspection of the drum, and if it is entirely normal then the diagnosis is otitis externa. However, in practice it can be very difficult to distinguish between the two conditions, either because the drum is not clearly seen, or because the inflammation of the canal associated with chronic otitis media is mistaken for otitis externa.

Topical application of antibiotics, and regular toilet hasten recovery in both conditions. (Do not be concerned about instilling topical antibiotics into the ear in the presence of a chronic perforation.)

Patients with otitis externa should be reviewed by their general practitioner within a week, and patients with chronic otitis media should be reviewed within the next couple of days by the ENT surgeons. It is a wise precaution to refer all patients with discharging ears in whom the drum cannot be adequately visualized if the history is suggestive of chronic otitis to the ENT surgeons.

Patients with a history of associated vertigo, and a positive fistula sign should be referred for an immediate ENT opinion.

Outcome

This patient had a large perforation of the ear drum on examination. He responded to aural toilet and Sofradex ear drops, and was symptom free at 10 days. Due to persisting hearing impairment he was advised to have a tympanoplasty.

Reference

Ludman, H. (1988) *ABC of Ear, Nose and Throat.* BMJ Publications, London

Case 41

A 34-year-old woman was advised to come to the Accident and Emergency department by her dentist. She had presented to him with a tooth abscess which he had drained. During the consultation she had confided in him that she had taken at least 16 paracetamol tablets during the past 24 h because of the intense pain. In the Accident and Emergency department the senior house officer obtained a further history. It transpired that in addition to those 16 tablets, she also admitted taking a further 10 tablets late the previous evening after a row with her boyfrined. She admitted to being under considerable stress. This was due partly to the pressure of her job, and partly to the fact that she recently discovered that she was pregnant. She did not want the pregnancy, nor did she want to continue seeing her boyfriend, but he was adamant that she should not have an abortion. It was over 3 months since her last period. Previously she had enjoyed good health, there was no history of previous psychiatric illness, self-harm, or serious medical illness.

On examination:

- Tearful
- Anxious
- Mental state examination was otherwise normal
- Blood pressure 100/65 mmHg, pulse 100/min
- Uterine size was compatible with a 12-week gestation
- Otherwise clinical examination was normal
- Beta-HCG was positive

Questions

1 What are the clinical features of a paracetamol overdose?
2 What is the mechanism of paracetamol toxicity?
3 What is your management in this case?

Answers

1 Paracetamol poisoning presently accounts for approximately 200 deaths/year. As few as 30 tablets (15 g) may prove lethal. Early clinical symptoms consist of nausea, vomiting and abdominal pain, which may be present within a few hours of ingestion, though typically patients are asymptomatic for the first 18 h or so. Within a day of ingestion early hepatic damage gives rise to right upper quadrant pain, though signs of acute hepatic necrosis with jaundice do not appear for 36–48 h. Encephalopathy usually becomes evident at approximately 72 h, with the patient initially drowsy (Grade 1), then confused (Grade 2), incoherent and agitated (Grade 3) and finally unresponsive to all but deep pain stimuli (Grade 4).

Altered consciousness within hours of ingestion is not a feature of paracetamol poisoning, and should suggest the presence of other toxic substances and/or alcohol.

However, delays in presentation are quite common after paracetamol overdose which may be partly due to the lack of early symptoms. A survey performed at one liver unit of 147 patients who were referred to them, found a median delay of presentation to their local hospital of 30 h.

Altered consciousness can be a feature in these patients who present late. Consequently it is important to include paracetamol poisoning in the differential diagnosis of altered consciousness and coma.

The patients who do die of paracetamol poisoning do so in liver failure approximately 5–7 days after ingestion.

Renal impairment is usually mild and consists of a transient rise in the creatinine and urea levels, though frank renal failure in the absence of severe hepatic damage has been described.

2 Paracetamol is inactivated in the liver by conjugation. In therapeutic doses 85% is conjugated with glutathione and sulphate and 10% is oxidized. Oxidation produces an intermediate metabolite, which subsequently undergoes conjugation with glutathione. When the system is overloaded, glutathione stores are depleted allowing build-up of the toxic intermediate metabolite. This hydroxylamine metabolite directly affects both liver and renal cells, giving rise to both hepatic and renal necrosis.

The aim of treatment is to raise intracellular levels of glutathione to mop up excess hydroxylamine metabolite. The most effective agent available is *N*-acetyl cysteine.

3 There are three aspects to the management of this woman.

a *Management of the acute overdose.* This patient presents with a history of ingestion of 26 paracetamol tablets, between 12 and 24 h previously. Gastric lavage is recommended within 4 h of ingestion and therefore would be unhelpful here. The serum paracetamol level should be estimated, along with the prothrombin time (the most sensitive early indication of liver damage). In addition: urea, creatinine and electrolytes; liver function test; blood glucose; blood gases and serum for toxicology.

The serum paracetamol level, when plotted on a standard concentration-against-time-chart will indicate whether a potentially toxic amount is present. If in the toxic range acetylcysteine should be started.

If the history is suggestive of an overdose of greater than 20 tablets (10 g) then acetylcysteine should be commenced immediately while the levels are awaited. The rationale behind this is that it can always be stopped if the serum levels are not in the toxic range.

Acetylcysteine should be given for levels in the toxic range within 24 h (though some authorities believe 36 h) of ingestion.

Adverse effects occur during the administration of acetylcysteine. These include nausea, vomiting, skin rash, hypotension and tachycardia.

Approximately 10% of patients will have an allergic response, and a few patients will have a full blown anaphylactic reaction.

For generalized mild reactions, the infusion should be interrupted, chlorpheniramine 10 mg i.v. administered and the infusion restarted running at a slower rate. Full blown anaphylaxis should be treated as stated on p. 88.

An individual's ability to handle a paracetamol overdose is variable and depends upon many factors including dose ingested, over how long, whether the patient vomited and the individual's rate of metabolism. Children, for reasons not clearly understood, appear to be able to tolerate paracetamol overdose much better than adults.

The following findings suggest severe liver damage and the patients should be discussed with the local liver unit.

i Early systemic acidosis, pH <7.3 at 24 h.
ii Rising prothrombin of 45+ at 48 h (over 100 is a very poor sign).
iii Early rising creatinine (300 mmol/l).
iv Rapid development of grade II encephalopathy (Grade III, IV are very poor signs).

b *Assessment of the patient's suicide risk.* Deliberate self-poisoning is very common, particularly in young females. The act is usually impulsive rather than premeditated, and commonly involves overdose of drugs such as benzodiazepines, analgesics or psychotropic drugs, and/or alcohol. The motivating factors behind such acts are often complex, though the majority of patients have no real desire to die. Actual suicide risk is highest in the elderly, where social isolation and depressive illness are common. Only a minority of these patients have a frank psychotic illness, though many patients have psychological symptoms.

Clinical evaluation of such patients includes:

i Assessment of intent – ask about the following:
- Is there an obvious precipitating cause, and has that now resolved?
- Were there signs of premeditation, with intricate plans, (e.g. precautions against discovery), and a suicide note?
- Does the patient still consider suicide as an option (suicidal intent)?
- Is the patient disappointed that she did not die?

ii Relevant past history – high risk categories for suicide include:

- Increasing age
- Social isolation (unemployed, widowers, elderly)
- Psychiatric illness
- Previous suicide attempts
- Family history of suicide
- Drug/alcohol abuse
- Major physical illness

iii Clinical assessment: the patient's mental stage should be assessed and in particular evidence of clinical depression or psychotic illness should be sought.

All patients should ideally be interviewed by a psychiatrist. Important further information may be obtainable from family members or the general practitioner. All patients with a risk of suicide will need to be admitted, for their own protection.

c *Consider the effect of the overdose on the pregnancy.* Further counselling on the potential risk to the pregnancy will be necessary. This should be performed by the general practitioner in consultation with the psychiatrist, the gynaecologist and the regional poison centre.

Outcome

This woman did not have a toxic serum level of paracetamol, nor did she have any alteration in her liver function tests or prothrombin ratio. After consultation with the regional poison centre it was decided that the prothrombin and liver function test should be repeated in 24 h. These too were normal.

As there was no medical reason to detain this woman, she was seen by a liaison psychiatrist who agreed with the assessment in the Accident and Emergency department that she did not constitute a high suicide risk.

She was discharged back to the care of her general practitioner with a letter explaining the nature of the episode, the blood levels, the psychiatrist's impressions and the need for further counselling.

Reference

Henry, J. and Volans, G. (eds) (1984) *ABC of Poisoning*. BMJ Publications, London

Case 42

A 54-year-old academic lifted a heavy box of books onto a table and suddenly developed excruciating central chest pain. The pain radiated up to his jaw and through to his back, and made him sweat and feel short of breath. Five minutes after the onset of the pain, he developed additional pain in his right buttock which radiated down his right leg and was associated with paraesthesia. His work colleague was shocked at his pale complexion and called an ambulance. He arrived in the Accident and Emergency department 30 min after the onset of the pain.

He was a heavy smoker and had a strong family history of ischaemic heart disease. A recent medical had failed to demonstrate any significant problem though he had been advised to stop smoking and lose weight.

On examination:

- Pale, sweaty, short of breath
- Respiratory rate 20/min, blood pressure 200/90 mmHg, pulse 110/min
- Jugular venous pressure elevated by 2 cm
- No bruits in the neck
- Auscultation revealed both systolic and diastolic aortic murmurs and a third heart sound
- There were bilateral basal crepitations and widespread wheezes
- Abdomen was soft, bowel sounds present
- All peripheral pulses were present
- Straight leg raising was painless to 90° bilaterally
- There were no focal neurological signs
- Electrocardiogram – tachycardia rate 110/min, there was 'T' wave inversion in the lateral leads I, AVL, V_6, but no other significant changes.

Questions

1 What is the differential diagnosis?
2 What is your immediate management?

Answers

1 Differential diagnosis

This man has acute left ventricular failure associated with an episode of chest pain, both aortic dissection or myocardial ischaemia are possibilities. This man, being a smoker, obese, and with a strong family history of ischaemic heart disease is at high risk for an ischaemic event. The nature of the pain is compatible with an acute myocardial infarction, though the electrocardiogram fails to demonstrate any obvious changes.

Dissection of the aorta should always be included in the differential diagnosis of any patient thought to have ischaemic pain, particularly if the pain radiates into the back, and is not associated with acute electrocardiographic changes. The sudden pain in the buttock would be unusual for a myocardial infarction though compatible with a dissection, and the recent onset of aortic regurgitation makes dissection the likely diagnosis.

With the increasing use of streptokinase and other thrombolytic agents, dissection should be considered and excluded early in the management of patients with chest pain.

2 Management

1 Relief of left ventricular failure

    a Sit patient up and give 60% oxygen via Venturi mask

    b Diamorphine 2.5–5 mg i.v. will be anxiolytic, aid dyspnoea and relieve pain

    c Frusemide 80 mg i.v.

    d Sublingual glyceryl trinitrate spray

    e Nebulized salbutamol for the wheeze

2 Control of hypertension

    a Nifedipine 10 mg (bitten and then swallowed)

    b i.v. nitrate infusion

3 Additional clinical signs compatible with dissection should be sought.

    a Blood pressure inequality between arms

    b Absent or diminished pulses

    c Bruits in the neck

    d Request an urgent chest radiograph – looking for mediastinal widening

Refer the patient to the medical team for angiography, contrast CT, or oesophageal echocardiogram.

Outcome

Dissection was thought to be a distinct possibility in this man and he was commenced upon an intravenous nitrate infusion to control his blood pressure while an aortogram was being organized. A repeat electrocardiogram demonstrated hyperacute anterior septal changes. Shortly after this he collapsed and died. At post mortem he was found to have a type 1 dissection of the aorta which had ruptured into his pericardium.

Further notes on dissection of the aorta

Dissection of the aorta is commonly misdiagnosed as an ischaemic episode, and should always be included in the differential diagnosis of any patient with anterior chest pain. Degeneration of the aortic media plays an important role in the pathogenesis of the condition, and there is a strong association with arterial hypertension. It is also associated with Marfan's syndrome, coarctation, and rarely pregnancy and cranial arteritis.

DeBakey classified dissection into three types:

Type 1 Starts in the ascending aorta, and involves the arch and descending aorta, that is it involves the whole of the aorta.

Type II Is confined to the ascending aorta alone.

Type III Is confined to the descending aorta.

Clinical features depend upon the site of the involvement (see below).

As with myocardial infarction, dissection tends to occur in men aged 40–70 years. The pain is most severe at the outset (in contrast to myocardial infarction which tends to build up over minutes) and is often described as 'tearing' or 'ripping' in quality. The pain may migrate (as it did in this man) as the dissection progresses, into the buttocks and down the legs.

The dissection may move proximally to involve the aortic ring giving rise to aortic regurgitation, or involve the coronary ostia on occasion giving rise to an associated acute myocardial infarction. This is typically an inferior infarct due to involvement of the right coronary ostium, as involvement of the left coronary is usually a terminal event. Extension of the tear into the pericardium gives rise to cardiac tamponade and a dissection of the descending aorta may rupture into the left chest. Involvement of the carotid arteries, or spinal arteries may give rise to the signs of a cerebrovascular accident or acute paraplegia which may give rise to diagnostic difficulties.

The majority of patients are known hypertensives and 50% will have evidence of long-standing hypertension, with left ventricular hypertrophy on the electrocardiogram.

The chest radiograph may be abnormal with evidence of widening of the mediastinum, or a localized bulge of the aorta. The diagnosis is made by arteriography or by CT scanning. Transthoracic echocardiography is not a reliable investigation to exclude dissection, though trans-oesophageal echo is useful.

Management is aimed at relief of pain, lowering the systolic blood pressure to 90–100 mmHg, confirming the diagnosis and early surgery.

Dissection of the aorta is often not diagnosed because the condition is not considered. The following case histories are typical.

Cautionary tales

A 68-year-old woman developed sudden pain between her scapulae which radiated down her back. The woman was admitted with a diagnosis of reflux oesophagitis made by the Accident and Emergency SHO which was changed to acute muscular skeletal pain by the admitting medical team. She died the next morning of her dissection.

A 57-year-old hypertensive male was admitted to exclude an infarct. Serial electrocardiograms and enzymes were normal. He was kept in hospital as his blood pressure was very labile. A further episode of chest pain which radiated to his jaw and through to his back occurred. Again there were no serial changes in his electrocardiograms or enzymes. Two days later, he died and a post mortem revealed a chronic dissection and an acute type 1 dissection.

Practice points

Always consider dissection in any patient with severe central chest pain, especially if:

a the pain radiates through into the back
b the patient is hypertensive
c the electrocardiogram is normal
d there is aortic incompetence or any signs compatible with the diagnosis
e loss of pulses (may be intermittent).

Reference

Camm, A. J. Cardiovascular disease in *Clinical Medicine.* (eds Kumar and Clark) (1st edn 1987). Baillière Tindall, London

Case 43

A 35-year-old woman presented with a 2-day history of a painful stiff knee. She could not recall any obvious trauma. She was also concerned that she might be pregnant as her last period had been 2 weeks late and unusually light. A full history revealed that she had been on holiday in Brazil with a girlfriend for a month and had returned from there 2 weeks ago. She had three episodes of unprotected intercourse while on holiday. There was no history of dysuria, vaginal discharge or lower abdominal pain. However, over the past 2 weeks she had had morning stiffness particularly affecting her knees and ankles. While abroad she had been well, without any diarrhoea or vomiting.

In the past she had no history of joint disease or other serious previous medical history.

On examination:

- Well
- Pyrexial 37.8°C

- Blood pressure 120/70 mmHg, pulse 90/min
- No rash
- Chest clear, cardiovascular system normal
- Abdomen soft
- Very swollen left knee, with obvious fullness in the parapatella fossae, and in the suprapatella pouch, not red, but warm
- Positive patella tap
- No localized tenderness
- Knee flexion very limited 10–70°
- No other joints involved
- Urine – clear
- Pregnancy test negative

Questions

1 What is the probable diagnosis in this woman?
2 How would you manage this patient?

Answers

1 Diagnosis

This woman presents with a monoarthritis. Common causes of an acute monoarthritis include:

a Septic arthritis: this is the most serious cause of an acute monoarthritis and should be excluded in all cases.
b Gout.
c Reactive arthritis.
d Degenerative arthritis/inflammatory arthritis.
e Bursitis and trauma.
f Miscellaneous: pseudogout, haemophilia, idiopathic etc.

a Septic arthritis

If left untreated septic arthritis is destructive, and can lead to total joint destruction within weeks. It presents as do other forms of acute monoarthritis, with an acutely swollen painful joint. Septic arthritis commonly affects the large weight-bearing joints of the lower limb particularly the knee. The most important diagnostic procedure is joint aspiration with joint fluid analysis and culture.

In adults the majority of episodes arise as a result of haematological spread from a transient bacteraemia, associated with a distant source of infection (urinary tract infection, skin sepsis, pneumonia), though penetrating wounds, joint aspirations and injections, and prosthetic joints account for a small number of cases.

The majority of cases of septic arthritis present with obvious signs and symptoms. The patient is systemically unwell, there is an acutely hot swollen joint, which may appear red, and muscle spasm in the flexors and extensors of the joint leads to a considerable decrease in the range of movements.

In the early stages of the illness both children and the elderly may have misleadingly subtle signs and typical signs of infection can be masked in patients on steroids.

Perhaps the commonest potential cause of septic arthritis seen by Accident and Emergency SHOs is that to the metacarpal phalangeal joints complicating a compound 'divot' fracture sustained by punching someone in the mouth.

The commonest organisms giving rise to septic arthritis are:

i *Staphylococcus aureus* (commonest in age range 2–15 years, and >40 years)
ii *Streptococcus* species
iii *Neisseria gonorrhoeae* (commonest cause in women 15–40 years)
iv Gram-negative organisms.

With the exception of *Neisseria*, many patients developing septic arthritis have an underlying predisposing cause. These include:

i Diabetes, cirrhosis, malignancy
ii i.v. drug abuse
iii Previous inflammatory joint disease, or surgery
iv Corticosteroids or immunosuppressants

In these patients there is a considerable morbidity and mortality.

Cautionary tale
A 50-year-old alcoholic professional musician presented with a systemic illness, an acute monoarthritis of his left knee and alcohol withdrawal. Aspiration of his knee revealed frank pus. Despite intensive treatment he died 8 days later.

Systemic gonococcal infection usually presents with a polyarthritis, tenosynovitis, and vesicopustular rash, though in 25% of cases the presentation is with an acute monoarthritis. Certainly, any otherwise fit woman presenting with an acute monoarthritis should be assumed to have a gonococcal arthritis until proven otherwise.

It is important to take cultures from many different sites at presentation to confirm the diagnosis because blood cultures and joint fluid are often negative on culture. With appropriate treatment, the prognosis is good, with patients seldom requiring arthrotomy, and the majority experience a quick and full recovery.

b Gout

The clinical presentation of gout especially in a large joint such as the knee can closely resemble that of septic arthritis. The joint is red, swollen, and acutely painful in both conditions. However, even in the presence of an overwhelming history of gout, joint aspiration and fluid analysis and cultures are necessary in all cases to exclude infection; as both conditions can occasionally coexist.

The diagnosis of gout is confirmed by finding characteristic intracellular, negatively birefringent needle-shaped urate crystals in the aspirate.

Seventy five per cent of all new clinical cases of gout present with pain in the metatarsal-phalangeal joint of the great toe and this is the typical way that patients with gout present to Accident and Emergency.

The clinical diagnosis of gout can be made when more than six of the following criteria are positive:

i   More than one attack of acute arthritis
ii   Maximum inflammation developed within one day
iii Monoarthritis attack
iv   Redness over the affected joint
v   Attack in the first metatarsophalangeal joint
vi   Unilateral tarsal joint involvement
vii Tophi
viii Hyperuricaemia
ix   Asymmetrical joint swelling on X-ray
x   Periarticular joint erosion on X-ray
xi   Joint fluid culture negative.

Treatment

When gout is confirmed by needle aspiration, the mainstay of treatment is rest and NSAIDs. The patient with large joint gout should be managed by a rheumatologist.

Do not be tempted to prescribe allopurinol, as not only may it increase the severity of the acute attack, it would not be indicated after a single episode of the disease.

Pyrophosphate crystals rather than urate crystals would suggest the diagnosis of pseudogout however, sepsis should again be positively excluded.

c Reactive arthritis

The precise aetiology of reactive arthritis is unknown. It is most likely due to an abnormal immune response to an infective agent in a predisposed individual (the majority of patients with reactive arthritis are HLA B27 positive). It usually affects the large joints of the lower limb. Commonly recognized triggers include:

i Sexually acquired reactive arthritis – perhaps associated with chlamydial infection.

ii Post dysenteric – following *Salmonella, Shigella, Campylobacter* and *Yersinia*.

iii Post viral – *parvovirus, coxsackie and Epstein-Barr virus*.

Again joint aspiration is essential to exclude septic arthritis.

d Degenerative and inflammatory arthritis

Degenerative arthritis, particularly of the knee is prone to give rise to recurrent sympathetic effusions. The history and X-rays should suggest the diagnosis, however, excluding septic arthritis is essential in all cases by examining the aspirate.

Inflammatory arthritis, such as rheumatoid, and psoriatic disease may present with an acute non-traumatic monoarthritis. There may be no clinical evidence of an underlying systemic disease in these patients, and again acute management involves joint aspiration to exclude sepsis, NSAIDs and a rheumatology outpatient appointment.

Long-standing rheumatoid disease is a predisposing factor for septic arthritis and any monoarticular flare up of the disease should be treated as septic until proven otherwise.

Bursitis

This woman presents with what appears to be an acute monoarthritis. Bursitis and trauma should always be considered when a patient presents with an acutely swollen knee.

A common condition which might be mistaken for acute monoarthritis of the knee is an inflammation of the prepatella or infrapatella bursas.

Inflammation of the bursa of the knee occurs most commonly in patients who do a lot of kneeling, hence the terms miners' and housemaids' knee.

There is localized tenderness, swelling and usually redness of the affected bursa. The knee appears swollen, and this is often mistaken for an effusion. Lack of fullness in the parapatella fossae and the suprapatella pouch and absence of a patella tap confirms that the inflammation is confined to periarticular structures. Movements of the knee are limited, but in contrast to acute arthritis the passive range of mobility is not as greatly affected as is the active range. Occasionally prepatella bursitis is associated with an effusion in the knee joint, and then septic arthritis should be excluded.

Trauma

As a haemarthrosis can simulate an acute monoarthritis a history of trauma should always be sought. Significant trauma is unlikely to be forgotten by the patient unless they had altered consciousness at the time, for example the patient was intoxicated, or had a fit.

However, even a history of significant trauma can be misleading. It is not uncommon for patients with proven septic arthritis to be able to recall an episode of recent trauma (see Cautionary tales, below).

2 Management

This woman presents with a monoarthritis. Given her history the diagnosis is most likely to be gonococcal arthritis.

The following investigations are necessary:

- Joint aspiration: urgent microscopy and Gram stain; culture; urgent polarized light examination.
- ESR: full blood count; blood cultures
- Swabs: urethral; high vaginal; cervical; pharyngeal; rectal.

The patient should be referred to the medical/rheumatology team in consultation with a genitourinary physician.

Outcome

Joint aspiration revealed an excess of polymorphs but no organisms, and blood cultures were sterile on culture. Cervical swab however grew the gonococcus. Within 48 h of being commenced upon penicillin, there was a significant clinical improvement.

Cautionary tales

A young athletic man with a history of repetitive episodes of injury to his knee, twisted his knee while on a 15 mile walk for charity. The next day his knee was swollen, and he presented to Accident and Emergency. He was treated for a sympathetic effusion for 2 weeks before the diagnosis of septic arthritis was made.

A two-year-old girl fell and twisted her ankle. She continued to play for the rest of the day albeit with a limp. The next day, however, she was walking normally. On the third day the ankle was swollen and she would not bear weight upon it at all. An X-ray revealed a small torus fracture of her distal fibula. She was treated with tubigrip. Four days later, now fractious, pyrexial and anorectic she still would not put any weight on that foot. A diagnosis of septic arthritis was confirmed at operation.

Practice points

1 Joint aspiration and analysis of the fluid is necessary in all cases of acute monoarthritis to exclude sepsis.
2 *Neisseria gonorrhoeae* should be considered the primary putative diagnosis in any sexually active female who presents with a monoarthritis.

3 Staphylococcal and other forms of septic arthritis are severely destructive if left untreated. There is usually an underlying chronic illness which predisposes to sepsis in these patients.

Patients typically present with an acute monoarthritis with severe limitation of movement.

4 An acute flare up of rheumatoid arthritis should be considered septic, particularly if the patient is on steroids.

Notes on joint aspiration

All major joints, except the hip can be aspirated in Accident and Emergency departments. Strict aseptic technique is necessary throughout the procedure. Contraindications to needle aspiration are:

1 Being unfamiliar with the technique
2 Infected overlying skin
3 The presence of a prosthetic joint
4 The hip joint

Reference

Huskisson, E. C. Chapter 8 in *Clinical Medicine*. (eds Kumar and Clark) (1st edn 1987). Baillière Tindall, London

Case 44

A 42-year-old man presented with a laceration to his scalp. He said that a work colleague had assaulted him in the office following an argument about drinking at lunch-time. They had a fist-fight and he felt that the laceration had been caused by his colleague's ring. He denied any loss of consciousnes and had felt fine since. He was currently taking medication for epilepsy, but had not had a fit for over a year. He denied any other injury, and there was no other significant past medical history.

On examination:

- Cooperative and alert
- Smelled of alcohol
- Glasgow coma score 15
- Higher cerebral functions intact
- No focal neurological signs
- A 4 cm long full thickness laceration was present over his left parietal region
- Ears and fundi normal
- There was no other evidence of injury

Questions

1 What further history would you want?
2 What is your management?
3 What are the indications for
   i Skull radiographs after head injury?
   ii Admission to hospital after head injury?

Answers

1 It is highly unlikely that the laceration could be caused in the fashion described. Patients who have sustained head injuries may be amnesic for the event, and will not be able to give an accurate account of the injury. Important additional history would come from a witness to the event, so his place of work should be contacted. They were able to describe on the phone, that the initial blow had knocked him to the floor, and he had caught the edge of the table on the way down. He had remained unresponsive for 20 s but he was not observed to fit. Five minutes later he appeared normal and his secretary telephoned for a taxi to take him to hospital. Clearly this additional information accounts for his laceration and the amnesia for the event.

Contacting witnesses is often easier than assumed and should be attempted when you feel the history is deficient. Also, an assessment should be made of the length of the post-traumatic amnesia. The patient, remembered the secretary phoning for the taxi and therefore the post-trauma amnesia was less than 10 min duration.

2 *Management*

i   Skull radiographs should be performed as the patient was rendered unconscious. Skull radiographs were normal.
ii The wound needs to be digitally explored and cleaned, and then sutured under local anaesthetic in a single layer with a monofilament 4/0.
iii Ensure antitetanus prophylaxis is adequate.
iv Re-examine the patient to ensure he is fit for discharge.
v   Provide head injury instructions and explain their relevance.
vi Try to contact a friend/relative who is able to escort the patient home.
vii Arrange follow up for removal of sutures in 7–8 days by the general practitioner.

Patients without a skull fracture who are awake and orientated, with normal higher cerebral function, without neurological signs or symptoms after a brief period of unconsciousness (i.e. less than 5 min), may be discharged home.

3 *Indications for skull radiographs after injury*

- Loss of consciousness of post-traumatic amnesia.
- Neurological signs or symptoms.
- Suspected base of skull fracture.
- Suspected penetrating injury.
- Significant scalp bruising.
- Those difficult to assess; due to alcohol intoxication, recent fit, children, including all children under the age of 1 year.

Note: A simple laceration is not an indication for skull radiographs.

Indications for admission after head injury are:

- Confusion or other depression of the level of consciousness at the time of examination.
- All fractures.
- Patients with neurological signs or persistent symptoms such as headache and vomiting.
- All patients with CSF leaks, or suspected fractures of the base of the skull.
- Patients who are difficult to assess, e.g. drunks, or high-risk patients who will have no supervision at home.

Notes

1 Post-traumatic amnesia with full recovery is not an indication for admission.
2 Patients sent home should be given written instructions about possible complications and the appropriate action to take. The relevance of these instructions should be explained to the patients/relatives.
3 Such written instructions should contain advice about common post-traumatic symptoms, including resting in bed until the headache settles etc. A sample is seen below.

Example of a head injury warning card (courtesy of *ABC of Major Trauma*)

(Accident and Emergency department tel: xxx xxxx)

This person has recently sustained a head injury and should be kept under regular observation every two hours for the first 24 hours. The person should be asked to tell you his or her name, where he or she is, the year, who you are, and should show you that he or she can move all four limbs normally.

If the person develops any of the following problems he or she should be brought back to hospital without delay:

1 Drowsiness or excessive sleepiness
2 Confusion or disorientation

3 Severe headaches, vomiting or fever
4 Weakness of any limbs or double vision
5 Convulsion, seizure or passing out
6 Discharge of blood or fluid from ears or nose

Reference

Driscoll, P., Skinner, D. and Earlham, R. (1991) *ABC of Major Trauma*. BMJ
  Publications, London

Case 45

A man aged 42 presented to the Accident and Emergency department
with palpitations. They had started abruptly after sneezing. Over the past
10 years he had regularly experienced similar palpitations every couple
of months. The episodes were short lived, and did not trouble him. Today's
episode had been prolonged, and he felt lightheaded, though he did not
experience any shortness of breath or chest pain. He admitted to being a
heavy smoker and to drinking at least 10 cups of coffee each day. There
was no history of ischaemic heart disease or thyroid dysfunction.

On examination:

- Well
- Pulse 180/min regular, blood pressure 125/70 mmHg
- No evidence of heart failure
- No signs of thyroid disease

The monitor revealed the rhythm shown below.

Rhythm strip: II
25 mm/s; 1 cm/mV

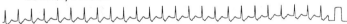

Questions

1 What is the rhythm?
2 What is your management?
3 What would your management be if the patient was taking atenolol
  100 mg o.d.?

Answers

1 The monitor demonstrates a regular 'narrow complex tachycardia'
(commonly called a supraventricular tachycardia). This is a non-specific

term, which strictly speaking applies to any tachyarrhythmia which originates above the ventricles with a QRS duration of less than 120 ms (three small squares).

Classifying these narrow complex tachycardias by their site of origin, they include:

- Sinus node: sinus tachycardia
- Atrium
  - atrial tachycardia (may be irregular)
  - atrial flutter (may be irregular)
  - atrial fibrillation (irregular)
- AV junction
  - atrioventricular re-entry tachycardia (AVRT, regular)
  - atrioventricular nodal
  - re-entry tachycardia (AVNRT, regular)

The commonest mechanism giving rise to a regular 'narrow complex tachycardia' is re-entry, though enhanced automaticity of myocardial cells outside the sinus node may well be the underlying mechanism in some arrhythmias. To understand the re-entry mechanism it is important to not to see the atrioventricular electrical conduit as a single entity, but two functionally separate pathways.

Normally both pathways conduct impulses synchronously to the ventricles. However, a premature atrial contraction may find one of these pathways refractory to antegrade conduction, as each pathway will have differing conduction velocities and refractory periods. The premature beat is then conducted to the ventricles by only one pathway, but is then able to re-enter the atrium by conduction retrogradely back up the other pathway, which is no longer refractory. This sets up a circuit motion, with each impulse not only activating the ventricles but also reactivating the atria, and so establishing the tachycardia. When the two pathways are wholly within the atrioventricular node it is known as a atrioventricular nodal re-entry tachycardia (AVNRT). In patients with an accessory pathway, e.g. Wolff-Parkinson-White syndrome, the mechanism is exactly the same, though in this condition the additional pathway is anatomically distinct from the atrioventricular node. The resulting tachycardia is known as a atrioventricular re-entry tachycardia (AVRT).

Patients with paroxysmal atrioventricular nodal re-entry tachycardias commonly have no evidence of ischaemic or valvular heart disease. The tachycardias tend to be recurrent, may present in infancy, and occur throughout the patient's life.

Many patients are asymptomatic during episodes, though shortness of breath, chest pain and hypotension are recognized particularly in those patients with pre-existing heart disease. The electrocardiographic characteristics are those of a narrow complex tachycardia, which is regular with a rate of 150–200 beats/min. Atrial activity is often not seen, as 'P' waves are concealed within the 'QRS' complex. Though, when they are seen, they are inverted and follow the 'QRS' complex.

For a detailed description of how to differentiate between different 'narrow complex tachycardias' from the surface electrocardiogram see Toff and Camm (1989).

2 The monitor reveals a regular narrow complex tachycardia. The patient is haemodynamically stable. Initial management should include:

- Reassurance
- Venous access (this is essential before attempting cardioversion)
- Twelve lead ECG
- Connect to a cardiac monitor

An electrocardiogram is important to exclude conditions such as atrial fibrillation with a fast-ventricular response which can appear regular on a monitor, as the treatment of atrial fibrillation and a atrioventicular re-entry tachycardia will differ.

Having confirmed that the rhythm is regular the response to vagal stimulation should be assessed. These manoeuvres attempt to increase vagal tone and thereby slow conduction through the atrioventricular node, interrupting the tachycardia circuit.

Vagal stimulation may not terminate the arrhythmia, but slow them, allowing 'P' waves to become more obvious.

Two forms of vagal stimulation are recommended.

i *Carotid sinus massage*: to be maximally effective this should be performed on the right carotid sinus with the patient supine. Gentle massage over the carotid pulse at the upper border of the thyroid cartilage over a 30-s period may be effective.
ii *Valsalva manoeuvre*: this can be performed by asking the patient to blow down the tubing of a sphygmomanometer and to sustain a pressure of 25–30 mmHg for 20 s.

(*Note*: Eye ball pressure is dangerous and should *not* be attempted, and swallowing ice is not very effective. In infants and children, however, a wet cold flannel on the face to provoke the diving reflex has been shown to be useful.)

If vagal stimulation is unsuccessful then drug therapy is recommended.

Drugs

i *Adenosine* has recently been made available and is now the treatment of choice for the rapid termination of supraventricular tachycardias. Given as a bolus dose it slows conduction through the atrioventricular node. This action may interrupt re-entry circuits involving the atrioventricular node, or aid diagnosis of 'broad' or narrow complex tachycardias by slowing the rate and therefore more clearly demonstrating atrial activity. Incremental doses of 3 mg, 6 mg and finally 12 mg are recommended, allowing each dose at least 2 min to work.

Common side effects include facial flushing, dyspnoea, chest tightness and nausea. At the time of conversion to sinus rhythm several benign, self-limiting arrhythmias have been documented. However, persisting, symptomatic sinus bradycardia may require a temporary pacing wire.

ii *Verapamil* 5 mg, given intravenously over a minute which can be repeated if there is no response in 5 min (up to 20 mg). If this fails to terminate the arrhythmia then the diagnosis should be reconsidered.

The most common side effect of intravenous verapamil is hypotension, and regular blood pressure monitoring should continue throughout the procedure. Hypotension may respond to calcium chloride i.v. Verapamil is contraindicated in patients taking betablockers as profound hypotension and bradycardias may occur, and in patients with digoxin toxicity.

Cardioversion If the patient is symptomatic, with chest pain, heart failure, or severe hypotension, cardioversion is the treatment of choice. The medical team and the anaesthetist should be called immediately.

On the return of sinus rhythm another 12-lead electrocardiogram should be performed to look for evidence of pre-excitation.

3 Treatment of a regular 'narrow complex tachycardia' when the patient is already on a betablocker consists of a small dose of intravenous betablockers such as atenolol 5 mg if adenosine fails. The major side effects of these drugs are hypotension and bradycardias. If you have no experience of using either of these drugs then request senior guidance.

Outcome

This man's tachycardia was unresponsive to vagal stimulation. However, he responded to adenosine 12 mg. A repeat electrocardiogram was normal and his potassium was 4.7 mmol/l. He was discharged home with an outpatient appointment to see the cardiologist.

Reference

Toff, W. D. and Camm, A. J. (1989) Differential diagnosis of narrow QRS complex tachycardia. *Hospital Update*, October, 758–770

Case 46

A Chinese man aged 25 presented with a 12-hour history of severe epigastric pain. The pain started suddenly and was constant but with sharp exacerbations which lasted 1–2 min. He was anorectic, nauseated and had vomited four times. The pain radiated through to the back but was not associated with eating or drinking and nothing relieved it. His bowels were normal and there had been no urinary symptoms. He had suffered with a similar pain 8 months ago which had lasted for 30 min only. There was no history of dyspepsia, or fat intolerance. He did not smoke, drink or take regular medications.

On examination:

- Apyrexial and in pain, sweaty
- Blood pressure was 120/70 mmHg, pulse 90/min
- Chest clear
- Epigastric tenderness and guarding
- Bowel sounds normal
- No hernias
- Rectal examination normal
- Urinanalysis normal

Questions

1 What is the differential diagnosis?
2 What investigations would you request?
3 What is your management?

Answers

1 Severe epigastric pain with vomiting can be caused by a number of different pathologies. Three which should always come to mind and which need to be actively excluded are:

a Biliary pathology – biliary colic/cholecystitis
b Perforated peptic ulcer
c Pancreatitis.

There can be considerable overlap in the symptoms and signs produced by these three conditions, and investigations are needed to confirm the diagnosis.

a *Biliary disease*. The clinical distinction between biliary colic and cholecystitis is usually straightforward. The pathological distinction however is not so clear and they probably represent clinical entities at either end of the same spectrum.

Biliary colic produces a poorly localized, sometimes colicky, but more often constant pain, in the epigastrium and right hypochondrium which may radiate through to the back or to the shoulder.

Signs are usually limited to tenderness and systemic upset is usually minimal. Associated vomiting is common and there may be a history of a previous attack.

The clinical diagnosis of acute cholecystitis is reserved for patients with systemic upset, fever and tachycardia, who have more pronounced abdominal signs, i.e. tenderness and guarding.

All patients should have a serum amylase estimation as pancreatitis may coexist. Ultrasound examination is helpful in confirming the diagnosis.

Biliary disease is more common in females (f/m ratio 2:1), and the majority are over the age of 50 years at presentation. The pain may be experienced solely in the right upper quadrant, exacerbated by inspiration, and by attempting to elicit Murphy's sign. However, diagnostic difficulty arises when the pain is poorly localized and felt vaguely in the right side of the abdomen, when it may have to be differentiated from appendicitis, or when it is felt across the upper abdomen.

A previous history of pain is helpful, especially self-limiting episodes of pain in the preceding 2 or 3 days.

b *Perforated peptic ulcer.* The pain with a perforation is of a sudden onset whereas that of pancreatitis tends to build over several hours. Patients are usually males, middle-aged or elderly and will look unwell. Movement exacerbates the pain and patients lie still. Any patient found rolling round the bed should lead you to suspect an alternative diagnosis.

Perforation occurs either on a chronic background of dyspepsia, or with a much shorter history where an additional factor is implicated, such as non-steroidal anti-inflammatory drugs. The patient initially has severe pain and the signs of localized peritonitis, which becomes generalized as the disease progresses. Free gas visible beneath the diaphragm will be present in 50–70% of patients with a perforation.

Occasionally, the perforation will be sealed by an omental plug giving rise to a much more confusing picture with localized signs.

c *Pancreatitis.* Very severe epigastric pain with recurrent vomiting is the hallmark of pancreatitis. Often there is a history of alcohol abuse, or biliary tract disease and many will give a history of previous, less severe attacks of similar pain. The pain is deep and boring in quality and radiates through into the back, and becomes more generalized as the disease progresses. Patients look ill and dehydrated, with a degree of hypovolaemic shock.

Localized signs in the abdomen are marked with widespread tenderness and guarding.

Serum amylase concentrations above 1000 i.u. are highly suggestive of the diagnosis, but values below this level do not exclude it.

Other conditions, e.g. generalized peritonitis can give rise to a significantly raised serum amylase (>500 i.u.) and should always be considered in differential diagnosis.

When the amylase is less than 500 i.u. pancreatitis is unlikely.

Perforated peptic ulcer may give rise to the same signs and symptoms and produce a rise in the amylase concentration, but this rarely exceeds 1000 i.u.

2 The following investigations should be performed in all patients with severe epigastric pain and vomiting:

(Results in this patient)

FBC	HB 14 WBC 7.6 PT 210
Urea and electrolytes	Normal
Amylase	192
Radiographs	
Erect chest	No free gas
Supine abdomen	No gall stones
Urinanalysis	No bilirubin, no blood
Group & Save	
BM Stix	7 mmol/l

When biliary disease is suspected and other pathologies have been excluded, ultrasound should be requested to confirm or refute the diagnosis.

3 Patients should be referred to the duty surgical team.

Outcome

The ultrasound in this patient demonstrated oedema of the gallbladder wall, with a single stone in Hartmann's pouch. He was admitted to hospital and had his gallbladder removed 72 h later.

Further notes on upper abdominal pain

Alternative diagnoses which should be considered in patients presenting with upper abdominal pain include:

a *Acute dyspepsia*. It is not uncommon to see young, usually male, patients who present with a short history of acute epigastric pain. There is often a history of heavy alcohol use, and many will have symptoms of acute gastritis, reflux, or peptic ulceration. The absence of abdominal signs, and typical symptoms enables these patients to be discharged back to the care of their general practitioners with a short course of H_2 antagonists and antacids.

Occasionally, patients present with severe symptoms and guarding. These patients should be admitted to exclude a perforation.

Cautionary tale

A 19-year-old man was admitted with acute epigastric pain which developed after a meal. He was acutely tender in the epigastrium with guarding. He was admitted for observation. An erect chest radiograph revealed the suspicion of free gas under the left hemidiaphragm, however it was not obvious whether this was a gastric air bubble. On attempting to pass a nasogastric tube the patient vomited a huge amount of food with complete symptomatic relief. On further questioning he had eaten eight pork pies for lunch!

b *Referred pain from the chest*

i *Ischaemic chest pain.* The pain associated particularly with acute inferior infarcts may be predominantly experienced in the epigastrium. An electrocardiogram is necessary in middle-aged and elderly patients particularly if the history is atypical.
ii *Basal pneumonia* and pericarditis should also be considered in the differential diagnosis.

Reference

Hamilton Bailey's Emergency Surgery, 11th edn. Wright, Bristol

Case 47

A man presented 24 h after being hit in the left eye with a cricket ball. He had an extensive periorbital haematoma and complained of blurred vision and intermittent double vision.

Visual acuity 6/12 left, 6/6 right.

Questions

1 What are the potential causes for his double vision?
2 What further examination is necessary?

Answers

1 Potential cause of diplopia after a blunt injury to eye are:

a Generalized impairment of ocular mobility due to the haematoma.
b 'Blow out' fracture of the orbit. This may involve the floor of the orbit and/or the medial orbital wall. Typically, 'blow out' fractures of the floor give rise to tethering of the inferior rectus muscle. This may give rise to diplopia on both upward and downward gaze.

The clinical signs associated with a blow out fracture are:

a Periorbital haematoma, with or without surgical emphysema.
b Marked bony tenderness of the inferior orbital margin.
c Paraesthesia in the distribution of the inferior orbital nerve.
d A subconjunctival haemorrhage inferiorly.

The diagnosis should be made clinically, as standard facial views often do not demonstrate the typical 'tear drop' herniation of the orbital contents into the maxillary antrum. Tomography or CT scan may be necessary to demonstrate the fracture. Patients should be referred to the ophthalmology team.

2 The eye should then be examined to exclude:

a Corneal abrasion or laceration.
b Hyphaema – bleeding in the anterior chamber gives rise to a cloudy anterior chamber acutely. As the blood settles it is clearly seen organized at the bottom of the anterior chamber. Recurrent bleeding may be massive and give rise to a secondary rise in pressure.
c Traumatic dilatation of the pupil due to rupture of the iris sphincter, or a tear at the iris periphery known as iridodialysis.

These injuries are often associated with damage to the posterior segment such as retinal oedema, retinal tear or vitreous haemorrhage. Urgent ophthalmology consultation is necessary.

Reference

Bron, A. J. and Davey, C. C. (1987) *The Unquiet Eye*. Glaxo Laboratories Ltd, Greenford

Case 48

The Accident and Emergency department receives a call from the local ambulance service. They inform you that they have just picked up a man in his twenties who was found unconscious on the pavement. He was seen to have jumped from a 30 ft (9.1 m) bridge.
No further information is available.

Questions

1 What injuries might you expect as a result of this fall?
2 What preparations would you make to receive this patient?

3 The patient is being wheeled into the department, lying prone on the trolley, as this was the position he was found in on the ground. What is your immediate management of this patient?

Answers

1 Various factors determine the injuries that will be sustained after a fall from a height. These include, the height above ground, the nature of the surface beneath, and what part of the body hits the ground first. Any fall from over 4 m above the ground should be considered sufficient to cause multiple injuries until clinical examination determines otherwise. The greater the height and the firmer the surface onto which the body impacts the greater the injury. Falls from the seventh floor onto concrete have been considered the highest level from which a person might survive. However, there are many documented cases of people falling from greater heights and surviving, but they usually landed upon a soft surface such as snow or water. There are even anecdotal stories of people surviving falls out of aeroplanes at heights above 18 000 feet (5486 m).

Compression–decompression and deceleration forces are responsible for the majority of injuries, and these forces can be transmitted along the axial skeleton giving rise to a typical distribution of injuries in people who, in particular, land on their feet.

Typical injuries of people falling onto their feet:

i A high proportion of lower limb fractures in particular to the calcaneum, ankle, tibial plateau and femur.
ii Axial transmission of energy frequently leads to crush fractures of the spinal column, often in the lumbar region but they can occur throughout the spinal column. Basal skull fractures have also been described following the upward thrust of the spine.
iii Injuries to vascular pedicles, most commonly that of the kidney, but also the hepatic veins and mesenteric vasculature are all well recognized.
iv Secondary impact, sustained when, after landing on their feet, the person falls forward etc. causes injuries to the upper extremities and to the face and head.

People falling onto their heads have a high incidence of craniofacial and cervical spine injuries, whereas compression and deceleration forces applied simultaneously to the chest, abdomen and pelvis can give rise to serious injuries, such as rupture of the aorta, a bronchus, major abdominal visceral and pelvic disruption.

2 From the history this patient should be assumed to have major injuries solely from the height of the fall. The fact that he is stated to be unconscious would signify the possibility of a serious head injury, profound shock or airway compromise.

The management of this patient demands a coordinated approach from the Accident and Emergency doctor, anaesthetist, general and ortho-paedic surgeon, radiographer and perhaps the operating theatre and blood transfusion, in short, a trauma team. All these specialists should be informed of the impending arrival of such a patient.

The resuscitation room should be prepared. All equipment which may be necessary should be conveniently positioned within the resuscitation area.

This will include:

- Anaesthetic machine: with airways, and fully working intubation equipment, suction.
- A rigid cervical collar.
- Intravenous fluids should be run through, and cannulas, blood bottles, and arterial gas syringe made readily available.
- The cardiac monitor should be switched on, with gel pads attached.
- Further equipment including:
     wound pads
     chest drains
     peritoneal lavage catheters
     urinary catheters/suprapubic catheters
     nasogastric tube
     pulse oximeter
  should all be available.
- All assembled staff should wear protective clothing including plastic aprons, gloves, glasses and a lead apron. The team leader, should allocate roles to all present so that multiple procedures such as intubation, venous access, observations and urinary catheterization can occur simultaneously rather than sequentially.
- Finally a large pair of scissors is necessary to cut through any clothes which are not easily removed.
- If everyone present is aware of their role and knows where vital equipment is to be found, the resuscitation can progress rapidly and smoothly.

The resuscitation of the multiply injured patient should follow the guidelines suggested by the American College of Surgeons (endorsed by the Royal College of Surgeons in England) in their Advanced Trauma Life Support Programme (ATLS).

1 **Primary survey** ⎞ identify and treat life-threatening injuries

2 **Resuscitation** ⎠ correct hypoxia and hypovolaemia

3 **Secondary survey:** thorough head-to-toe examination

4 **Definitive care:** a structured treatment plan

(1 and 2 occur simultaneously.)

3 *Initial management.* The initial management includes the primary survey and active resuscitation. The principles of which are found below.

As the patient comes into the department it is important that you take control of the situation.

Assessment

Talk to the patient. 'How are you?' A good positive response, 'oh yes I'm fine thank you', not only tells you that the patient has been very lucky, but that their airway is patent, the blood pressure is adequate to perfuse the brain normally, and, although a major secondary complication of a head injury is not excluded, it excludes significant primary brain injury.

When there is no response at all, as in this patient, immediate attention should be directed to the airway. To manage the airway and to protect a potentially injured cervical spine the patient should be log rolled into the supine position. Taking control of the head and maintaining in line immobilization, the patient should be gently lifted over onto his back, with the help of at least three additional persons, one taking the chest, one the pelvis, and one the legs. By orchestrating this movement, the head needs only to rotate through 90° to assume the neutral position, this combined with in line immobilization is highly unlikely to exacerbate any cervical injury.

Airway with cervical spine control. The airway should be cleared with suction and patency maintained with a 'chin lift' manoeuvre and if tolerated an oropharyngeal/nasopharyngeal airway.

Patients who are apnoeic need assisted ventilation via a cuffed endotracheal tube and 100% oxygen. Those who have low respiratory rates, i.e. <10/min need assisted ventilation.

Respiratory rates >10/min and <30/min require supplemental oxygen 60% via Venturi mask.

Respiratory rates >30/min, having ensured that the airway is patent a search for a life-threatening chest injury must be made.

Cervical spine. While maintaining the airway, the cervical spine should be immobilized with a rigid cervical collar which prevents rotational movements as well as flexion and extension. Care should be taken during manipulation of the airway not to move the cervical spine. Alternatives to using a rigid collar are: constant in line immobilization exerted by a member of staff or securing the head with elastoplast across the forehead onto the table either side, and sandbags placed on either side of the head to prevent rotation.

Breathing. The respiratory rate is a very underestimated observation and frequently not recorded. Rates above 30/min may indicate life-threatening chest injuries. These include:

- Tension pneumothorax
- Massive haemothorax
- Open pneumothorax
- Large flail segment of chest wall with underlying pulmonary contusion

A brief examination of the chest should be aimed at specifically excluding these conditions. Observation of chest wall movement may indicate decreased excursion on one side or paradoxical motion associated with a flail segment. Surgical emphysema, and fracture crepitus, would indicate chest wall injury, and unilateral hypoventilation may indicate an underlying pneumothorax.

The clinical presence of a pneumothorax with a respiratory rate of greater than 30/min should be taken as evidence of tension, as the other signs typically associated with an expanding pneumothorax, such as tracheal deviation, engorged neck veins, and pulsus paradox can be difficult to elicit particularly when there is associated hypovolaemia.

Therefore a clinical pneumothorax and respiratory distress (respiratory rate > 30/min) = tension pneumothorax.

Immediate relief of the tension is necessary. A 20-ml syringe attached to a cannula should be inserted into the second intercostal space in the midclavicular line on the affected side. Confirmation of a pneumothorax is evidenced by the easy aspiration of air. If present, disconnect the syringe leaving the cannula in place and a rush of air will be heard. This converts a tension into a simple pneumothorax. A chest drain should be inserted once the patient is stabilized. Absence of air implies that the diagnosis is incorrect, the cannula should now be removed. There is a 10–20% chance that this procedure will create a pneumothorax, (particularly if the patient is being artificially ventilated) and this should be borne in mind as the resuscitation continues.

An open pneumothorax needs to be covered with air-tight material such as cling film, or Opsite and a chest drain inserted to drain that hemithorax immediately. Open pneumothoraces are potentially lethal as air can be preferentially sucked into the chest through the chest wall defect, and not down the trachea.

The rare massive haemothorax (>1500 ml), if present, will need to be drained immediately by a large bore chest tube.

Successful prompt relief of such conditions, helps correct hypoxia and leads to a considerable improvement in the patient's condition.

Circulation. Stop any obvious external haemorrhage, with direct pressure exerted by sterile gauze; no tourniquets or artery clips.

Cold, clammy peripheries, with a delayed capillary return (>2 s) implies hypoperfusion as does a significant tachycardia and hypotension. Two intravenous cannulas should be inserted in either antecubital fossa, blood taken for crossmatch and fluid given. For patients with signs of hypoperfusion a fluid bolus of up to 2 l (crystalloid and colloid) should be given. Remember that the early signs of hypovolaemic shock can be difficult to detect especially in the young and under-transfusion is much more common than over-transfusion. For persisting hypotension after the 2 l bolus, blood should be given (uncrossmatched if necessary) and immediate plans to take the patient to theatre should be made.

The patient should be attached to the cardiac monitor, and the vital signs checked regularly. A urinary catheter should be inserted if the signs of urethral injury have been excluded. A urine output of 1 ml/kg/h is normal for an adult and indicates adequate tissue perfusion and therefore adequate fluid replacement.

Blood gas estimations should be made.

Dysfunction. A brief neurological examination is necessary. Check the pupils, are they equal and both reacting to light? Is the patient alert, spontaneously opening his eyes, or responding to verbal commands, if so can he squeeze your fingers with both hands or wiggle his toes? Is he only responding to painful stimuli, if so do all four limbs move equally? Is he completely unresponsive to all stimuli, from such information the Glasgow coma score can be calculated.

It is important to continue to document the score, along with changes in the other observations, as significant changes may occur during the initial resuscitation.

Exposure. If not already completed the patient should have all his clothing removed. The only safe way to do this is by cutting them off with scissors. Remember however the patient should be covered with blankets to conserve heat, immediately the examination is complete.

Radiographs

Radiographs of the chest, pelvis and cervical spine should be requested as soon as the patient arrives, and should be taken during the initial resuscitation.

The chest radiograph should be requested first, to exclude potential causes of hypoxia not suspected during the initial survey. Remember that supine films may not easily demonstrate blood or air in the pleural spaces. The pelvis is a potential source of life-thereatening haemorrhage and is often associated with major intra-abdominal injury. It is important to know about severe disruption of the pelvis early.

If properly immobilized any neurological damage associated with an injury to the cervical spine should not be further exacerbated during the resuscitation, but remember intubation, and movement of the patient, may jeopardize this situation. A lateral cervical spine radiograph demonstrating C1 to the upper border of T1 is imperative. It can be difficult to visualize all the cervical vertebrae at the first attempt, especially in a heavily-built patient, and it is not uncommon for several attempts to fail. In order to increase your success rate, before taking the first lateral cervical film, with the help of three other people attempt to pull down the shoulders to enable you to demonstrate the cervicothoracic junction. One person should maintain in line immobilization of the neck, one person should pull down on each upper arm, and the fourth person should stabilize the trolley. If unsuccessful, a swimmer's view, or a 30° oblique film can be useful to demonstrate the lower cervical spine.

The initial resuscitation is now complete, and you should be well on the way to correcting any hypoxia and hypovolaemia. However, you are far from arriving at a diagnosis. If you have stabilized the patient it is now necessary to determine the full extent of the injuries, by performing a thorough head-to-toe examination of the patient (secondary survey). Further investigations whether radiographs, peritoneal lavage, ultrasound or CT scan will be determined by the clinical impressions gained during this thorough survey.

Further management should be determined by the team leader.

Practice points

1 The mechanism of injury can give you a very good indication as to the amount of energy dissipated during the accident and therefore an idea of the extent of the injuries to detect and be found.
2 An integrated and simultaneous approach by a trauma team is necessary.
3 The commonest causes of death from major trauma are hypoxia and hypovolaemia. Conditions giving rise to these complications should be corrected early.
4 The initial assessment therefore is directed to identifying and treating life-threatening injuries.

Remember

- Airway with cervical spine control
- Breathing
- Circulation
- Dysfunction
- Exposure

Reference

Driscoll, P., Skinner, D. and Earlham, R. (eds) (1991) *ABC of Major Trauma*. BMJ Publications, London

Case 49

A 6-year-old girl was brought by her parents, because within the last hour she had accidently swallowed the plastic top of a felt tip pen. There was no history of choking, coughing, difficulty in breathing or cyanosis and the child had been asymptomatic since.

The parents were very anxious, and requested that an X-ray should be taken. They had thoughtfully brought along a similar plastic top from another felt pen. It measured 2.5 cm long by 0.7 cm wide.

On examination:

- Child was well
- No respiratory distress, respiratory rate 17/min
- No recession, or use of accessory muscles
- Chest clear, no wheezes or stridor
- Pulse 90/min, blood pressure 90/60 mmHg
- Abdomen soft
- Bowel sounds normal
- Otherwise examination was normal

Questions

1 What is your general management of ingested foreign bodies?
2 What is the management in this case?

Answers

1 General management

The management of children who have ingested a foreign body depends upon (a) the foreign body in question, and (b) the site of the foreign body at presentation.

The foreign body

The list of objects swallowed by children at some time or another is exhaustive. The majority are inert and harmless and if they have passed to the stomach, can be confidently expected to be passed in the stools within one week. However, it may take as long as 4 weeks for some foreign bodies to be passed.

The narrowest part of the gastrointestinal tract is at the level of the cricopharyngeus, and any foreign body which does not become impacted will usually be able to circumnavigate the remainder of the gastro-intestinal tract.

Even potentially dangerous objects such as 'open' safety pins, razor blades, and thermometers have all been passed uneventfully once they have reached the stomach. Recently much attention has been focused upon button batteries which have been associated with a number of fatalities due to their corrosive nature, but again virtually all cells which reach the stomach will pass spontaneously without any symptoms or complications. (See below for specific management of ingested button batteries.)

The site of impaction

In the majority of children, the foreign body will be in the stomach or beyond at presentation. The lodgement of a foreign body in the upper or lower respiratory tract or the oesophagus carries particular risk.

Inhaled foreign bodies. Inhalation of foreign bodies occurs particularly in infants. Although the vast majority of such foreign bodies will end up in the bronchus (usually the right) some will lodge in the trachea or larynx. A history of coughing, choking or respiratory distress occurring at the time of inhalation should always be sought.

As so often happens though, the infant is not observed when the incident happened, and therefore a history of sudden respiratory difficulty, hoarse cry stridor, or wheeze in a previously fit child should always raise the possibility of an inhaled foreign body.

In some children the inhalational episode goes unrecognized and the child may present days, weeks or months later with recurrent chest infections, or recent onset of wheezing.

Oesophageal impaction. Impaction in the oesophagus gives rise to chest discomfort and an inability to swallow. In young children this is often manifest as excessive drooling, and the child will refuse liquids and solids.

Clinical examination should always include a thorough examination of the chest, looking in particular for stridor, wheeze, signs of differential air entry, or asymmetrical chest movement. The ability of the child to drink should always be assessed, and an inability to do so would suggest oesophageal impaction. Tenderness and focal signs in the abdomen should be excluded.

Radiology

Not all children will need an X-ray.

The following will:

- Any child with a history on examination compatible with inhalation should have a chest X-ray. Radiopaque foreign bodies, if inhaled, will be visible, and radiolucent foreign bodies may give rise to suggestive radiographic changes. These include focal collapse, compensatory emphysema, and air trapping or a combination of these features.

- Any well apyrexial child who suddenly develops stridor should have a lateral radiograph of the soft tissues of the neck. However, this should be done under controlled circumstances with an anaesthetist, a paediatrician and an ENT surgeon present.
- Any child with the symptoms of oesophageal impaction.
- Any radiopaque foreign bodies, particularly if they are potentially dangerous such as button batteries and safety pins.

A single 'chin down' radiograph should suffice in infants as the chest and upper abdomen will be included on the single film. Older children will need two radiographs, one of the chest and one of the abdomen.

There is no point in performing X-ray examinations on children who are asymptomatic, in whom inhalation has been excluded, when they have ingested innocent or radiolucent foreign bodies.

Admission policy

The following are indications for admission to hospital:

1 Children who are thought to have inhaled a foreign body, either from the history or the examination.
2 Children with symptoms of oesophageal impaction or a confirmed oesophageal foreign body.
3 Children with abdominal pain and/or vomiting.
4 Children who have ingested potentially dangerous foreign bodies such as button batteries or 'open' safety pins.

Button batteries

The fatalities associated with button batteries have been associated with oesophageal impaction. Once they pass to the stomach most will pass spontaneously without complication. However, some batteries leak, or disintegrate leading to the potential of local corrosive damage and systemic mercury poisoning. For this reason, children should be referred to the paediatric team for admission. H_2-antagonists should be given, to reduce gastric acid secretion, and thereby potentially decrease the change of battery cell disintegration secondary to corrosion. Metaclopromide, if the battery is still in the stomach, will promote gastric emptying and laxatives such as lactulose will hasten transit time.

Discharge policy

The majority of children can be discharged.

The parents should be reassured that the majority of foreign bodies will pass spontaneously within the next 4 weeks.

There is no need to do repeated radiographic examination of the child at weekly intervals to check the progress of the foreign body. Parents should, however, be advised to return immediately if the child develops abdominal pain, persistent vomiting, or evidence of bleeding.

2 Management in this case

This child has ingested an inert plastic top. The history or examination is not suggestive of potential inhalation, and certainly from the size of the top one would expect significant symptoms if it had been inhaled.

In the absence of symptoms suggestive of impaction in the oesophagus, the child should be asked to swallow a sip of water. Patients with impacted oesophageal foreign bodies will rarely be able to do this without symptoms. If this is performed easily then the parents should be reassured that the top has passed at least as far as the stomach and should therefore pass without any problem. As the plastic top is radiolucent, an X-ray is unnecessary and this should be explained to the parents.

Although there will be no need for the child to be reviewed again routinely, they should return if the child develops symptoms.

Outcome

The parents were reassured and the child was discharged.

Reference

Kiely, B. and Gill, D. (1986) Ingestion of button batteries: hazards and management. *British Medial Journal,* **293,**

Case 50

A 46-year-old company director was brought in 'unconscious', to the Accident and Emergency department by a work colleague who was obviously drunk. He had called the ambulance as he had found the patient covered in vomit and unrousable, on the pavement outside a pub. They had been celebrating excellent half-yearly sales figures, when wanting a breath of fresh air, the patient had left the pub. When he had not returned 20 min later, the colleague had gone to look for him. He found him at the bottom of the three steps leading down from the pub.

The only other information the colleague could give was that the man was divorced, lived alone and had recently been given the 'all clear' at a company medical. The colleague apologized to the Accident and Emergency staff for causing such inconvenience, admitting that they had probably had 'one too many' this time. The ambulance men could add little to the history though they had noticed that the patient was opening his eyes initially, but now this had stopped.

On examination:

- Smelled of alcohol and vomit
- Spontaneous respiration 10/min, pulse 60/min regular, blood pressure 140/100 mmHg
- Chest clear
- Occipital haematoma with a scalp laceration
- No other evidence of trauma

Neurology:

- Pupils equal and reactive to light
- Ears normal, fundi normal
- No neck stiffness
- No eye opening to painful stimuli
- Groaned only to painful stimuli
- Feeble attempt to remove noxious stimuli by both hands
- Each foot withdrawn when nail bed pressure applied
- There were no focal neurological signs
- No needle marks
- BM stix 7 mmol/l

Questions

1 What is your working diagnosis?
2 What is this patient's Glasgow coma score?
3 What is your management?

Answers

1 The working diagnosis must be head injury with suspected intracranial damage and a potential cervical spine injury. Never assume that alteration in conscious level is due to alcohol until all other causes have been excluded. The mechanism by which he sustained this head injury is not known as it was not witnessed. It is easy to assume that a man, intoxicated, trips, falls down the steps and bangs his head outside a pub, thereby sustaining a head injury and a possible cervical spine injury. However, other possibilities should be borne in mind; was he assaulted? hypoglycaemic? did he have fit? has he been taking drugs with the alcohol? The clinical examination should be thorough to look for evidence of other precipitating factors.

2 His Glasgow coma score is 8. Patients with a score of 8 or less are by definition, in coma. The score is calculated using the scale below:

Eye opening		Best motor response		Verbal response	
Spontaneous	4	Obeys commands	6	Orientated	5
To command	3	Localizes pain	5	Confused	4
To pain	2	Normal flexion	4	Utters words	3
None	1	Abnormal flexion	3	Utters sounds	2
		Extensor	2	None	1
		None	1		

The lowest score possible is 3 in a patient who has no response whatsoever to any stimuli, and the highest is 15 in a normal individual. One should be proficient at using this system to score all head injuries, as it conveys a much more precise picture of the clinical state when talking to colleagues and neurosurgeons, than do vague terms, such as semicomatose. It also allows early recognition of changes in the clinical state.

If you find it difficult to remember the scale you should carry a copy on a small piece of card in your pocket acting as an 'aide mémoire'.

3 *Urgent management of a patient with a severe head injury*
(The initial assessment should follow the sequence as in Case 48).

- This patient is in coma with evidence of a head injury, the anaesthetist, and duty surgeon should be called immediately.
- The airway should be managed throughout the resuscitation and 60% oxygen administered via Venturi mask.
- The cervical spine should be immobilized using a rigid cervical collar.
- Any potential life-threatening chest injury should be identified and treated immediately (unlikely, given the story, but he may have been stabbed).
- The circulation should be assessed, venous access should be established, and the patient attached to the cardiac monitor.

  Blood pressure, pulse, respiratory rate and the Glasgow coma score should be measured every 15 min. Hypotension should be treated with intravenous fluid, an an extracranial source of bleeding suspected.

  BM stix estimation for exclusion of hypoglycaemia.

  Consider giving naloxone if there is any evidence of opioid drug abuse.

  Measure arterial blood gases.
- Catheterize and pass a nasogastric tube (NB: if there is fresh blood in the nostrils, pass an orogastric tube).
- A full head-to-toe examination should then take place. This should include digital exploration of the occipital wound, for a fracture or foreign body and a systematic examination of the whole body for signs of injury, focal neurological signs, needle marks etc.
- Radiographs of the cervical spine, and skull should be requested. Remember a lateral film of the cervical spine should include C1 down to the upper border of T1.

Skull films are not necessary if immediate CT head scanning is available and should not delay transfer to the neurosurgeons for CT scanning.

- Benzylpenicillin 1 mega unit i.v. and sulphadimidine 1 g should be administered for compound skull fractures, or suspected base of skull fractures. Tetanus status should be considered deficient and immuno-globulin i.m. should be administered. (Alternative antibiotic regimens include ampicillin, flucloxacillin and metronidazole.)
- Control initial seizures with intravenous diazepam (5–10 mg); exercise great care, as patients with acute neurological damage can be very sensitive to benzodiazepines which can precipitate a respiratory arrest.

Phenytoin 250 mg as a bolus over 10 min, and then 500 mg over the next 4 h should be prescribed to prevent further seizures. The patient should be attached to a cardiac monitor during the administration of phenytoin. Up to 20 mg/kg may be given if the patient continues to fit.

Guidelines for consultation with a neurosurgeon

The following patients should have a CT head scan, and be discussed with the regional neurosurgeons:

1 Patients with a fractured skull in association with:
   i Confusion
   ii Glasgow coma score <15
   iii Focal neurological signs
   iv Fits
   v Persisting neurological symptoms, e.g. persistent vomiting
2 Coma continuing after resuscitation (Glasgow coma score <8), in the absence of a skull fracture.
3 Deterioration in the Glasgow coma score of 2, or developing neurological signs.
4 Confusion or neurological disturbance persisting up to 8 h in the absence of a skull fracture.
5 Compound depressed skull fractures.
6 Suspected base of skull fracture – evidenced by leak of cerebrospinal fluid from the nose or ears, bilateral orbital haematomas, haemotympa-num or frank blood from the ear, retromastoid haematoma.
7 Penetrating head injuries – missiles, gun shots etc. The use of mannitol at 0.5–1 mg/kg (i.e. 250–400 ml of a 20% solution for adults) is a powerful osmotic diuretic and may be life saving. Its use is only recommended after consultation with the neurosurgeons.

Indications for intubation in patients with severe head injuries

1 Unprotected airway
   No gag reflex to oropharyngeal suction
   Excessive blood or vomit in pharynx

2 Inadequate ventilation or hypoxia
    Inadequate respiratory rate <10/min
    $P_aO_2 < 9\,kPa$ when breathing air or $P_aO_2 < 13\,kPa$ in a patient on supplemental oxygen
    $P_aCO_2 > 5.3\,kPa$
3 Therapeutic hyperventilation to control raised intracranial pressure. Again this should be done in consultation with the neurosurgeons.

Outcome

There was no obvious evidence of a precipitating cause for the fall, or sign of any other external injury. He was haemodynamically stable, and digital exploration of the scalp laceration revealed a fracture. Standard cervical spine radiographs failed to demonstrate the C1–T1 junction, however a swimmer's view demonstrated it beautifully. There was no obvious abnormality on the cervical spine films. He was given benzylpenicillin and sulphadimidine for the compound fracture, tetanus immunoglobulin and tetanus toxoid.

His condition was then discussed with the neurosurgeons who suggested elective hyperventilation, and mannitol 1 mg/kg.

A CT scan demonstrated an occipital contusion and generalized cerebral oedema. He was managed with an intracranial pressure monitor, and made a slow and incomplete recovery.

Practice points

1 Never attribute coma to alcohol excess until all other causes have been excluded.
2 Remember to safeguard the airway, and cervical spine as a priority in all serious head injuries.
    Call a senior anaesthetist and surgeon immediately.
3 Always exclude hypoglycaemia and consider drugs in the differential diagnosis, as these are reversible.
4 The Glasgow coma score should be calculated frequently during the resuscitation.
5 Discuss all serious head injuries with the neurosurgeons.

Further notes

In any Accident and Emergency department on a Friday or Saturday night there will be a number of intoxicated patients who have fallen over as a consequence of drinking alcohol and arrive semicomatose. The vast majority of such patients will just be drunk, without significant head injury and will sleep off the alcohol in the department, wake up, be very ungrateful, and leave in the morning. These are typical 'heart sink' patients, who need careful assessment and continual observation if serious intracranial pathology is not to be missed.

Galbraith (1976) stated that it is a common mistake to attribute the depression of the conscious level to alcohol intoxication rather than head injury, resulting in the delay in the diagnosis of some intracranial haematoma.

Remember the incidence of intracranial haematomas in unconscious patients after head injury with a skull fracture is 1:4 and 1:32 without a skull fracture.

The following are necessary:

1 Ensure vital functions are stable.
2 Exclude hypoglycaemia.
3 Consider drug overdose and give naloxone to patients with suspicious signs.
4 Any patient with an obvious history of head injury, or signs of such e.g. scalp haematoma, should be managed as the patient in the above case. All patients need to be examined thoroughly for signs which would be incompatible with alcohol intoxication, e.g. focal neurology.
5 All patients should have skull radiographs. Any patient with a fracture should be referred directly to the surgical team for a CT scan.
6 Alcohol level: measured by breath test, or blood testing is helpful only if the level is absent or very low suggesting that the alcohol plays no part in the altered consciousness. High levels do not necessarily mean that the alcohol is the cause of the coma, as habitual drinkers can be quite awake in the presence of extremely high alcohol levels.
7 Regular observations with repeated estimations of the Glasgow coma score are necessary every 15 min. Most patients however drunk will usually respond to a maximal painful stimulus.

A typical response to a painful stimulus is:

a try to remove the stimulus (5)
b swear at you (3)
c open their eyes (2)

giving them a Glasgow coma score of 10. The trend with acute alcohol intoxication is a slow gradual improvement over a number of hours. Deterioration in this score over a period of time or no response at all to maximal stimulus should be reviewed with suspicion. If in doubt call for a senior opinion.

Whether these patients are nursed in the Accident and Emergency department, observation or general ward will depend upon local facilities. However, these patients should not be sent home until they have recovered.

References

Galbraith, S. (1978) Misdiagnosis and delayed diagnosis in traumatic intracranial haematoma. *British Medical Journal*, **1**, 1438–1439

Driscoll, P., Skinner, D. and Earlham, R. (eds) (1991) *ABC of Major Trauma*. BMJ Publications, London

Case 51

A man aged 62 years presented with chest pain. He was a taxi driver and had a heated exchange with a garage owner when he realized that his cab would not be ready on time. During the argument he was aware that he had chest discomfort which felt as though someone was tightening a belt across his chest. The tightness progressively became more noticeable and uncomfortable. He stopped arguing and sat down. He was not able to catch his breath, and he was very sweaty. The tightness was now a pain across his chest, but it did not radiate to his throat, jaw or arms. Fifteen minutes after it had started the pain subsided and he felt back to normal. The garage owner had called the ambulance. On the way to hospital he was asymptomatic, and was only persuaded to stay on arrival, by the ambulance men. In the past he had been diagnosed as having ulcerative colitis 10 years ago, but this had given rise to only occasional intermittent diarrhoea since it was well controlled with salazopyrin. He was a smoker, and many of his family including his mother and father had died from ischaemic heart disease.

On examination:
- He looked well
- Apyrexial
- Pulse 84/min, blood pressure 160/95 mmHg
- No evidence of cardiac failure
- Chest was clear
- Heart sounds normal
- Abdomen was soft
- ECG revealed sinus rhythm but no acute changes compatible with ischaemia or infarction

Question

What is your management of this patient if:

a This is his first attack of chest pain?
b He is known to have ischaemic heart disease, and has had two myocardial infarctions previously 5–8 years ago. He frequently has self-limiting pain like this when emotional.

Answer

This man gives a good clear history of ischaemic type pain which was short lived, lasting 15 min and was precipitated by emotional upset. Management of patients who present with angina will differ depending upon the history, examination and ECG.

a If this was his first attack of chest pain the patient needs intensive medical treatment as an inpatient. He should be treated as having unstable angina, as the next attack of acute ischaemia could occur at any time and may result in myocardial infarction or death. The rationale behind this management decision comes from a better understanding of the pathophysiology of coronary artery occlusion. Clinical angiographic studies show that a high proportion of patients with recent onset angina have segments of coronary arteries with ragged outlines of the intima and intraluminal filling defects. These are thought to indicate plaque fissuring and intraluminal thrombus. Plaques are lipid rich extracellular collections of mainly cholesterol compounds which lie encapsulated in the intima. They may break through the endothelium and become exposed to the luminal contents acting as a nidus for thrombus formation.

The thrombus may grow to occlude the lumen and then propagate distally, or lyse and allow the plaque to reseal. The process is dynamic, the situation changing over hours and days, and may end in total occlusion of the artery and consequently myocardial infarction or sudden death.

All such patients with recent onset of ischaemic type chest pain should be referred to the medical team on call.

b Although myocardial infarction can occur without chest pain, or with chest pain which is very short lived, the majority of recognized acute infarctions are associated with prolonged chest pain (more than 15 min). This patient with known ischaemic heart disease has stable symptoms. Patients with long-standing heart disease have time to develop a collateral circulation and thereby decreasing the possibility that 15 min of chest pain signifies myocardial damage. If the electrocardiogram does not demonstrate any changes compatible with acute ischaemia or damage, and complications of acute ischaemia such as heart failure are excluded the patient can be discharged home. He should be advised to return immediately if symptoms return.

The clinical differentiation between an attack of angina and evolving myocardial infarction is not always possible. Useful clinical points to help distinguish are:

Favour angina

- Precipitated by exercise, emotion, etc.
- Terminated by rest, relaxation etc.
- Eased within 1–2 min by sublingual glyceryl trinitrate
- Less than 15 min duration. (An arbitrary time scale, but has some clinical relevance.)

Favour myocardial infarction

- Pain starts at rest, or if precipitated by exercise or emotion, it is not terminated by rest or relaxation
- No effect of sublingual glyceryl trinitrate
- Generally more severe than their typical angina and more prolonged in duration.

Note: All patients with probable ischaemic type chest pain should be given aspirin 150 mg to chew while being assessed in the department.

Outcome

This man had a history of stable angina. He commonly developed chest pain in emotional situations, and he was not surprised that he had had an attack during this argument.

He was discharged back to the care of his general practitioner with a letter, and an outpatient appointment to see the cardiologist. He was commenced upon a betablocker (atenolol 100 mg) in addition to the isosorbide dinitrate.

As he was a taxi driver he was also advised not to drive until he had seen the cardiologist (see Medical Aspects of Fitness to Drive).

Further notes

Unstable angina

Unstable angina is a clinical diagnosis made on the history. Patients with the following features should be considered as unstable.

1 Increasingly severe and prolonged episodes of chest pain provoked by decreasing amounts of exercise.

Figure 18   Clinical diagnosis of unstable angina

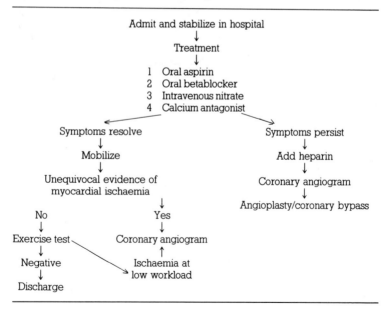

2 Angina of recent onset (last 4 weeks).
3 Prolonged (>15 min) chest pain at rest.

Patients with unstable symptoms are at risk from myocardial infarction and sudden death. The management of such patients is detailed in Figure 18.

References

McMurray, M. and McLenachan, J. (1990) Unstable angina. *Prescribers' Journal*, **30**, 165–172
Medical Aspects of Fitness to Drive. Medical Commission on Accident Prevention

Case 52

A 79-year-old woman was brought in by ambulance having been found at home in a collapsed and unresponsive state. The only history available was that while preparing to go out shopping she had suddenly called out, vomited and collapsed to the ground. The vomit was described as being 'coffee grounds', by the ambulance men.

On examination:

- She was unresponsive. Not cyanosed
- Sweaty
- Tachypnoeic 30/min
- Tachycardiac 130/min (palpated at the femoral)
- Cold extremities with absent distal pulse
- Capillary return delayed
- Unrecordable blood pressure

Questions

1 Which of the following conditions count account for these physical findings?

   a Pulmonary embolus
   b Pancreatitis
   c Myocardial infarction
   d Massive gastrointestinal bleeding
   e Tension pneumothorax
   f Cerebral haemorrhage

2 What is your immediate management?

Answers

1 (a) True
  (b) False
  (c) True
  (d) True
  (e) True
  (f) False

The patient has presented with acute shock. Hypovolaemic shock precipitated by a massive gastrointestinal bleed would be a distinct possibility, but pancreatitis would not produce this degree of shock so catastrophically. By limiting venous return, both pulmonary embolus and tension pneumothorax could produce this picture. However, one might expect the patient to be cyanosed.

Cardiogenic shock associated with a myocardial infarction is another possibility which could give rise to this clinical condition. However, an intracerebral event causing sudden collapse usually gives rise to a slow respiratory rate, and a bradycardia not the signs of shock.

2 When presented with a patient who is acutely ill, without adequate history to form a structured management plan rely on basic principles.

i Summon help immediately.

ii **Airway**: ensure the airway is clear, maintain it with a chin lift manoeuvre and a oropharyngeal/nasopharyngeal airway, and given 60% oxygen by Venturi mask.

iii **Breathing**: examine the chest to exclude positively a tension pneumothorax. Remember the signs of respiratory distress (respiratory rate >30/min) and clinical evidence of a pneumothorax should be taken as indicative of this condition. The additional signs of mediastinal shift, and engorged neck veins if present confirm the diagnosis. If present urgent treatment is necessary (see Case 30).

Crepitations and wheeze would be indicative of pulmonary oedema secondary to a cardiac event or pulmonary embolus.

iv **Circulation**: establish venous access with two large cannulas, (14 gauge) take blood for crossmatch and baseline investigations and run in 2 l of fluid (Hartmann's, Haemaccel), as quickly as possible.

v Examine the abdomen for evidence of a pulsatile mass in the epigastrium, rigidity and perform rectal examination for melaena or fresh blood.

Quickly examine the scalp and the patients back for obvious signs of injury.

vi Reassess vital signs and functions to document any improvement or deterioration.

Further history

With the administration of fluid her clinical condition improved rapidly. She regained consciousness and responded verbally. She was able to give the following history:

She had felt well that morning, had breakfast, then while preparing to go out she had suddenly developed excruciating epigastric pain which radiated through to the back, and that is the last thing she recalled. She denied having any chest pain or breathing difficulty. Her only recent complaint was pain in her buttock and right thigh when she walked. In the past she had been treated for hypertension and took tablets for arthritis. She denied any dyspeptic symptoms and there had been no history of haematemesis or melaena.

Clinical examination now revealed:

- Sweaty, cold peripheries. Respiratory rate 24/min
- Jugular venous pressure not visible
- Blood pressure 90/60 mmHg, pulse 110/min
- Clear chest
- Abdomen – distended and tender. No masses or guarding
- ECG – tachycardia, ST depression in leads I, AVL, V5 and V6. No changes of acute infarction
- Chest X-ray normal. No evidence of pulmonary oedema, no free gas beneath the diaphragm
- BM stix – 8 mmol/l

Questions

3 What further management is necessary?
4 What is the diagnosis?

Answers

3 i Further fluid replacement, and blood when available. Central venous pressure measurement. A central venous pressure line should be inserted to monitor fluid replacement in a patient with a potentially poor cardiac reserve.

ii Urine output – a catheter needs to be inserted.

iii Arterial blood gases – to ensure adequate oxygenation and ventilation.

iv Ultrasound examination of the abdomen.

4 The diagnosis is most likely to be a ruptured aortic aneurysm. Epigastric pain radiating through to the back associated with profound hypovolaemic shock is a typical presentation. The acute mortality of this condition is high

(perioperative mortality 36–60%); the majority of patients die. The absence of a pulsatile mass does not exclude the diagnosis. Such a mass can be difficult to palpate in an obese, or hypotensive patient. The pain she has been experiencing in her buttock and thigh is suggestive of claudication secondary to aorto-iliac disease.

Gastrointestinal haemorrhage is not associated with excruciating pain. Rarely a perforated ulcer may erode through an artery, giving rise to pain and hypovolaemic shock. The shock associated with a large pulmonary embolus may improve dramatically as the clot moves more distally, however, the history and clinical signs make this an unlikely diagnosis. The electrocardiogram reflects the tachycardia but is otherwise normal for a woman of her age. There is no evidence of a major cardiac event.

Outcome

Laparotomy revealed a large retroperitoneal haematoma associated with a rupture of the aorta. She died during an attempt to repair it.

Practice points

1 The incidence of abdominal aortic aneurysm is increasing, and rupture/leak of an aneurysm should be included in the differential diagnosis of any elderly patient with abdominal pain.
2 A pulsatile abdominal mass is not an invariable finding, and can be missed when the patient is obese, hypotensive or has significant guarding of the abdominal muscles.
3 If a patient has a pulsatile mass clinically, and abdominal pain, always assume that the aneurysm is responsible.
4 Aortic aneurysm should always be excluded in the elderly presenting with renal colic, or back pain.
5 Ultrasound is the investigation of choice.

Further notes

The incidence of aortic aneurysms is increasing. When patients present with abdominal pain, a pulsatile abdominal mass, and shock the diagnosis is straightforward. However there are many atypical modes of presentation.

Pryor (1972) studied 44 patients admitted to hospital who presented with a ruptured abdominal aortic aneurysm. In this study only 14 patients were correctly diagnosed at presentation, in a further 14 the diagnosis was made later on the ward, one was diagnosed at laparotomy for suspected appendicitis, and 15 were diagnosed at post mortem.

Although 18 patients presented with abdominal pain, pulsatile mass and shock, the aneurysm was felt to be intact in four of them, which led Pryor to invoke the old adage, when a patient with an abdominal pulsatile mass develops abdominal pain, always assume the aneurysm is responsible.

On rupture of an aneurysm immediate fatal exsanguination does not automatically follow, as the haematoma can be contained in the retroperitoneal structures. There are reports of patients who have chronically leaked for a period of over 3 months. The leaking of blood into the retroperitoneal structures can give rise to back pain, diagnosed incorrectly as an acute lumbar disc, pancreatitis, or renal colic. In fact, the presentation with ureteric colic is so well recognized that some authors suggest that any patient over the age of 55 presenting with such symptoms should be scanned to exclude an aneurysm.

Cautionary tale
A 70-year-old man with a history of chronic back pain suddenly collapsed with acute back discomfort. He was pale, sweaty with a blood pressure of 100/60 mmHg. A lateral radiograph of the back revealed a crush fracture of L2, about which there was a lot of discussion as to whether it was old or not. The radiographs also revealed the calcification in the wall of an 8 cm aneurysm. This was not noted at the time. The patient then began to complain of abdominal pain, at which time the pulsatile mass was discovered.

With increasing age, and increasing tortuosity of the aorta, aneurysmal dilatations can be found at sites quite remote from the midline, raising the possibility of a kidney tumour, psoas abscess or even obstructed hernias. I have certainly been misled by an aneurysm which I diagnosed as a vascular renal mass.

An ultrasound scan is the investigation of choice when diagnostic difficulty arises. In the absence of a skilled operator, a plane supine, abdominal radiograph is useful and is often diagnostic. Diagnostic accuracy, however, depends upon the observer looking for the calcification in the aneurysm which is usually associated with a large soft tissue mass, and for loss of the psoas shadow.

References

Pryor, J. P. (1972) Diagnosis of ruptured aneurysm of abdominal aorta. *British Medical Journal*, **2**, 735
Murie, J. (1989) Editorial. *Hospital Update*, **15**,

Case 53

A man presented with sudden painless loss of vision in his right eye. He described the episode as if someone had pulled a curtain over his vision.

In the past two days he had noticed several black spots floating in the vision of that eye.

On examination:

- Visual acuity – he could only perceive the difference between light and dark
- Visual fields revealed intact peripheral vision in his upper temporal quadrant
- There was loss of the red reflex, and his retina could not be seen
- There was an afferent pupil defect.

Questions

1 What is the diagnosis?
2 What other conditions may present as painless loss of vision?

Answers

1 *Retinal detachment.* This man gives a good history of a retinal detachment. This condition may be traumatic but most commonly it occurs spontaneously in short-sighted people. Typically there is loss of peripheral vision, but visual loss may be profound if the macula is involved. Vitreous floaters and flashing lights can be a warning of imminent retinal detachment. These are caused by traction on and tearing of the retina due to collapse of the vitreous gel.

Any patient presenting with a recent onset of floaters or flashing lights should be referred, as 5% will have a retinal tear, which will need repair.

2 Other causes of painless loss of vision:

Vitreous haemorrhage. A vitreous haemorrhage presents with sudden loss of vision, with loss of the red reflex and an inability to visualize the retina. It can occur secondary to a retinal tear or proliferative diabetic retinopathy. Most haemorrhages clear spontaneously within a couple of days allowing specialist treatment of the underlying cause.

Retinal artery occlusion. This most frequently occurs secondary to embolization in patients with arteriosclerotic disease. In any patient over 55 years of age cranial arteritis should be excluded from the history and ESR estimation. The red reflex is present, and there is typically pallor of the retina, and constricted arterioles. Branch occlusion may occur, which may be overlooked by the inexperienced observer. Ophthalmology referral is necessary.

Retinal vein occlusion. This is more common than retinal artery occlusion. Loss of vision may not be complete, and a reasonable visual acuity maintained if there is a branch occlusion. It is common in hypertensives, diabetics and patients with hyperviscosity syndromes. The red reflex is present, and the retina is usually covered with many flame-shaped haemorrhages.

Little can be done about the acute process, but review by the ophthalmologist is necessary.

Outcome

With pupil dilatation a large retinal detachment was obvious which involved the macula. The inferior nasal retina was uninvolved accounting for the findings on testing the visual fields.

Reference

Bron, A. J. and Davey, C. C. (1987) *The Unquiet Eye.* Glaxo Laboratories Ltd, Greenford

Case 54

A 33-year-old woman with mild asthma presented with severe difficulty with breathing. It had started suddenly with chest tightness and an inability to take a deep breath. She quickly became increasingly distressed with the symptoms.

On examination:

- Tearful
- Pulse 100/min, blood pressure 110/70 mmHg, no paradox, respiratory rate 20/min
- Respiratory pattern, short shallow breaths, interspersed with very deep breaths
- Chest – good air entry, no wheeze
- Peak flow 490 l/min

Question

What is the diagnosis?

Answer

The diagnosis is hyperventilation syndrome. Hyperventilation is a complex condition, which may be precipitated by a variety of organic and psychological conditions. The term implies that the patient is 'over breathing', that is breathing in excess of their physiological requirements. This, however, may have a therapeutic value in patients for example with a metabolic acidosis.

Symptoms can be acute, with patients often presenting to the Accident and Emergency department, or more chronic in nature leading to long-term morbidity.

Conditions which may give rise to hyperventilation include:

- Anxiety and depression
- Panic attacks
- Phobic states, e.g. agoraphobics
- Severe pain
- Mild asthma
- Pulmonary emboli
- Aspirin overdose
- Factitious

Acute hyperventilation gives rise to easily recognizable symptomatology. (This is in contrast to the sometimes bizarre symptoms provoked by chronic hyperventilation.)

Common symptoms are:

- Fear
- Panic
- Inability to take a deep breath
- Unsteadiness
- Syncope
- Loss of consciousness (uncommon)
- Paraesthesia – around the mouth, and in the limbs
- Chest pain – atypical, brief lancinating pain, usually in the left submammary region
- Sympathetic over stimulation – tachycardia, dry mouth, tremors

The diagnosis is often suggested by the demeanour of the patient who is in the throws of an acute panic attack. The respiratory pattern is irregular, with periods of hyperventilation. Tetanic spasm of the fingers and wrist may be apparent. The history and examination should attempt to exclude a precipitating organic cause in the first instance, e.g. aspirin overdose, asthma, pneumothorax etc.

Management

1 Treat any underlying cause.
2 Patients normally respond to strong verbal reassurance. It is rarely necessary to resort to re-breathing from a paper bag.
3 In phobic states and panic attacks sedation with a benzodiazepine may occasionally be necessary.

4 Arterial blood gases. These demonstrate the hypocarbia, and a respiratory alkalosis. It also excludes a metabolic acidosis.
5 On resolution of the symptoms. Controlled hyperventilation, with patient breathing at a rate of 30/min for 3 min reproduces the symptoms. This confirms the diagnosis and helps to reassure the patient about the nature of their symptomatology.
6 Patients should be referred to their general practitioner for continued management.

Reference

Gardner, W. and Bass, C. (1989) Hyperventilation in clinical practice. *British Journal of Hospital Medicine,* **41**

Case 55

A homeless 72-year-old man was found unresponsive by the police in his cardboard box beneath the railway arches. He was well known to the department, being a frequent attender with problems usually associated with alcohol abuse. (He was in fact currently under regular review for pretibial laceration which required regular dressings.) There were no witnesses at the scene nor any empty bottles of alcohol or tablets. Records from previous attendances revealed phenytoin prescriptions for long-term epilepsy, alcohol abuse, and evidence of chronic self-neglect. No other information was available.

On examination:

- Airway clear
- Respiration, normal pattern 10/min, pulse 70/min regular, blood pressure 130/70 mmHg
- Chest clear
- Abdomen soft, bowel sounds normal
- General appearance dirty and unkempt
- Laceration to right shin – healing, and not infected
- No stigmata of liver disease
- Head, evidence of two old lacerations
- No eye opening to pain
- No verbal response to pain
- Localized painful stimuli and attempted to remove the noxious stimuli
- Pupils 3 mm, reactive to light
- Doll's head eye movements absent
- Oculovestibular responses absent
- Corneal reflexes absent

- Gag reflex intact
- Normal tone in limbs, reflexes brisk and symmetrical
- Flexor plantar responses

Questions

1 What is the emergency management?
2 What is the Glasgow coma score?
3 Where is the lesion?
4 What are the possible diagnoses?

Answers

1 See Appendix

2 Glasgow coma score

Glasgow coma score is 7.

3 Site of lesion

Widespread cerebral hemispheric and brainstem involvement secondary to a metabolic cause.

4 Diagnosis

The finding of normal pupillary responses in a patient with absent oculocephalic, and oculovestibular responses is highly suggestive of a metabolic cause of coma. A combination of alcohol and phenytoin toxicity could produce this picture. However, with the two lacerations to his scalp intracerebral damage needs to be excluded, e.g. a subdural haematoma. A CT scan was normal. Many drugs can produce coma in overdose and the commonest ones are listed below.

- Benzodiazepines
- Alcohol
- Opioids
- Barbiturates
- Anticonvulsants
- Tricyclic antidepressants
- Anticholinergics
- Phenothiazines

Alternative diagnoses that should be entertained in this man should include liver failure and Wernicke's encephalopathy.

Hypoglycaemia should be excluded.

Any patient with a history of alcohol abuse who presents in coma should be given thiamine 100 mg i.v., to protect against or treat Wernicke's encephalopathy.

Outcome

This man had high serum levels of both alcohol and diazepam. His clinical condition gradually improved over 48 h when he took his own discharge.

References

Plum, F. and Posner, J. B. (1980) *Diagnosis of Stupor and Coma*. F. A. Davis Co., Philadelphia
Springings, D. and Chambers, J. (1990) *Acute Medicine*. Blackwell Scientific Publications, Oxford

Case 56

A police officer requests a statement on a patient whom you saw a month ago after an assault.

Questions

1 How do you prepare a police statement from a casualty card?
2 When may a statement be released to the police?
3 What else should you do and know about its preparation and the release of information to the police?

Answers

1 Preparation

Preparing a statement from the clinical notes is a necessary part of the work of an Accident and Emergency department. It is helpful to use a standard format each time this is done. An example is found below.

Specimen statement

I am a registered medical practitioner currently employed as a casualty officer at St Elsewhere's Hospital.

The patient, John Doe, was brought to the Accident and Emergency department of St Elsewhere's Hospital at 23:35 on 10 December 1990 after an alleged assault. He gave the history that he had been kicked and punched about the head but denied any loss of consciousness, nausea, vomiting or visual disturbance.

I examined him and recorded that he was alert and orientated and that his general condition was satisfactory. I found the following injuries:

a A 4-cm jagged laceration to the right side of the forehead, running from the right eyebrow towards the hairline. The wound divided the full thickness of the soft tissues, exposing the underlying bone. The surrounding 5 cm area was swollen and bruised.

b A left-sided black eye.

c An area of tenderness and swelling some 5 cm in size to the left side of the back of the head.

d Superficial scratches and abrasions to the palms of both hands.

The patient's laceration was cleaned and closed under local anaesthesia with a total of 6 stitches. A vaccination was given to prevent tetanus and Mr Doe discharged at 01:15 on the 11 December 1990 with head injury instructions.

Notes

This statement should be typed rather than handwritten, giving you the opportunity to write the statement in peace and quiet rather than dictating it to a police officer; it also allows for greater legibility and sense of professionalism, and enables a photocopy to be retained in the department.

The statement should be completed on the appropriate form (no.991A) with your personal details completed at the top. The police statement should be signed and the signature witnessed. A claim form (no.459) for the appropriate fee should also be completed and submitted with the statement.

2 Release

This statement may be released to the police on the receipt of the patient's signed informed consent. It is the responsibility of the police to provide this – but many departments have appropriate consent forms that patients may sign, which are then kept with the notes, so that the return of these statements may be expedited.

If consent is not provided, the notes and the relevant casualty officer may be subpoenaed to attend court.

3 Further information

When preparing statements write concisely and accurately in layman's rather than medical terminology. The court does not wish to be baffled by science, and simple terms such as a black eye rather than a periorbital haematoma are more appropriate. Always attempt to record measured wound sizes and be as correct as possible in your description of injuries using accurate terms such as lacerations or abrasions or bruises.

Casualty officers are expected to produce statements relating to the factual findings of their examination. The patient's history is not strictly relevant, as it is hearsay, although it may be included to explain the subsequent management such as loss of consciousness in head injuries dictating the need for skull X-rays. Opinions are not generally required and should not be expressed without senior guidance.

Always ensure that copies of your statements are retained. If you are required to give evidence in court, ensure that your original notes are also available for you to consult. Should you have to prepare a statement on a patient seen in your department, but not by you, ensure that this is made quite clear. A useful form of words is as follows: 'Dr Jones, the casualty officer who interviewed and examined Mr Doe, was employed as a locum and is no longer working in this department. This statement has therefore been prepared from the records made at the time of Mr Doe's attendance'.

Case 57

A female child aged 15 months was brought by her mother having had a 'fit' at home. The child had been well until 15:00 when she suddenly developed a temperature and became irritable, refused tea and Calpol. At 19:00 she suddenly became rigid, turned blue, and then commenced shaking all over. The whole episode lasted 2 min. Afterwards she was drowsy and floppy. The mother had called for the ambulance. Previously the child had been well save for recurrent ear infections. Birth history was normal, and she appeared to be developing normally. The mother was single and lived with her two other children (aged 4 and 9) in a flat.

On examination:

- Flushed, pyrexial 38.4°C
- Irritable, screamed when examined
- Right ear drum red and bulging, left, normal
- Throat normal
- Chest clear
- Abdomen soft
- Neck stiffness impossible to assess

While a urine bag was being placed on the child, she suddenly became stiff, cyanosed and her eyes rolled up. Then she began to shake all over.

Questions

1 What is your immediate management?
2 What is the probable diagnosis?
3 What are the indications for admission after a fit?

Answers

1 *Immediate management*

a *Maintain and protect the airway*
The infant should be placed in the lateral semiprone position head down.
Excess secretion should be removed from the pharynx.
Oxygen via mask should be supplied.
A nasopharyngeal airway inserted if tolerated.

b *Terminate the fit*
Completely undress the infant.
Administer rectal diazepam 0.5 mg/kg (alternatively 5 mg for a child aged 1–3 years and 10 mg for children >3 years).

c Exclude hypoglycaemia with a BM stix.

d Cool the child with tepid sponging and a fan.

Rectal diazepam is easy to administer, though it may take several minutes to terminate the fit. If unsuccessful the options available are:

i If venous access is readily achieved give i.v. diazepam (0.25 mg/kg).
ii Paraldehyde 0.1 mg/kg, either rectally or i.m. into the buttocks.

The paediatric team should be called if the fit is not terminated by the above measures. Persistent fits not controlled with adequate doses of diazepam, should be controlled with phenytoin 15–20 mg/kg as an i.v. infusion over 20 min. Phenytoin is made up with 0.9% saline and infused at a rate <1 mg/kg/min. The infant should be attached to a cardiac monitor during the administration.

Note: neither diazepam nor phenytoin should be given intramuscularly. If phenytoin fails the anaesthetist should be called and thiopentone administered.

2 The most likely diagnosis is a febrile convulsion, precipitated by right otitis media. Convulsions are frightening to witness, and many parents feel their child is going to die. Febrile convulsions occur from 6 months to 5 years, with the highest incidence between 9 and 20 months. They are common, affecting 2–3% of all children. It is thought, that the rapid rise in the temperature is more important than the ultimate temperature. Between 30 and 40% of children will go on and have a further febrile convulsion in the future.

Poor prognostic signs for epilepsy are:

- First febrile fit greater than 30 min duration
- Focal features
- Repeated fits in the same illness
- Followed by transient or persistent neurological abnormalities
- Those with a family history of epilepsy or evidence of pre-existing abnormal development.

Management in the Accident and Emergency department should be primarily concerned with controlling the airway, then the fit and excluding hypoglycaemia. The history of a fit in this child is fairly typical. Children and infants do not froth at the mouth or bite their tongues and therefore fits have to be differentiated from breath-holding episodes and reflex anoxic or vasovagal attacks.

3 All children with a first febrile convulsion should be admitted to hospital for observation irrespective of whether a focus of infection can be found. The majority of febrile fits are associated with non-specific infection or upper respiratory tract infection, however, meningitis should always be considered. Children under the age of one year (and many believe 18 months) are subjected to a full septic screen, including lumbar puncture as meningitis may be present without localizing signs.

Outcome

Rectal diazepam (5 mg) controlled this second fit. She was admitted to hospital. Meningitis was excluded by examination of the cerebrospinal fluid and she was commenced upon amoxycillin for right otitis media. She was discharged home after 48 h. The mother was given a supply of rectal diazepam (Stesolid) and instructions on what to do if a fit was to recur at home.

Reference

Lissauer, T. (1981) Convulsions. Paediatric emergencies. *Hospital Update*, July, 741

Case 58

A 10-month-old baby girl is brought to the Accident and Emergency department by her mother late one evening with bleeding from her mouth. Her mother gives the history that she had placed the child on the bed, while getting her changed, and left the room to collect an article from the adjacent bathroom. She heard a cry and returned to find the child lying on the floor beside the bed. Mother is aged 19, a single-parent and living in bed and breakfast accommodation near the hospital. The child was admitted some 3 months previously following an unwitnessed fall from the bed. Although there was no definite loss of consciousness on that occasion, a skull X-ray was performed, which was initially thought to show a fracture. The child was therefore admitted and discharged the next day after overnight observation when the radiologists felt that the presumed fracture was a vascular marking.

Clinical examination revealed an alert, playful child whose only apparent injury is a torn frenulum, which is not actively bleeding.

Questions

1 What are your concerns?
2 What would your management be?

Answers

1 The clinical finding of a torn frenulum is suggestive, though not pathognomonic of non-accidental injury. The injury occurs most frequently as the result of a blow to the mouth, or when a child is feeding and a spoon or other implement is pushed forcibly against the lips and upper teeth. Injury to the frenulum may occur if the child falls, striking its lip across a rigid surface such as the edge of a table or chair and usually such a clear history can be elicited.

In this case the fall was unwitnessed and occurred through lack of supervision, but the mechanism of a fall from a bed to a carpeted floor is not compatible with the injury sustained. Further features in the history which may alert you is the previous similar injury and the nature of the social circumstances in a young and possibly socially isolated mother.

2 A full and detailed history of the episode and of the child's past history should be taken, paying particular attention to any inconsistencies in the story. The child should be undressed and a full examination carried out to exclude any evidence of other injuries.

The critical decision with an injury which is incompatible with the history or any other suggestion of non-accidental injury, is whether to admit the child to the paediatric ward at the time of initial presentation. This enables background information to be gathered, from social services, from the general practitioner and health visitor, or from the nursery or any school the child may attend. Observing the child on the ward may diffuse problems at home, allow assessment of the relationship between mother and child and most critically, bring the child into a safe environment.

Admission is therefore the safest option, either on the basis of the severity of the injury, or if there is real concern that the child remains at risk at home.

Where the suspicion of non-accidental injury is not high, but has been raised, the decision regarding admission or discharge should be made by a senior doctor either from the Accident and Emergency department or from the Paediatric unit and you should discuss the case with them. Unless admission is clearly appropriate, in which case the child and her mother should be offered a bed as rapidly as possible, the senior doctor should assess the child personally before deciding to discharge. It may be more appropriate to arrange for an early outpatient follow-up within a few days, thus retaining contact with the family and gathering appropriate information during the interval.

Further notes

The commonest mistake is failure to suspect the possibility of non-accidental injury and to accept each history at its face value. In Accident and Emergency departments a senior doctor or nurse with special paediatric experience should review all cards of the under 16s, relaying information about attendance back to the general practitioner or school nurse. Checking the Child Protection Register for all children attending from their catchment area identifies those children who have previously been considered at risk, and increases the level of suspicion. The attendance in Accident and Emergency departments of this particular group of children must be passed onto the appropriate Social Services department with responsibility for them. Many such children are brought to Accident and Emergency departments with often trivial injuries, because their parents wish those injuries to be accurately documented at the time, rather than face questioning by Social Services in retrospect.

Case 59

A man returned home from the cinema to find his 32-year-old flatmate suddenly confused. Three hours previously at supper he appeared entirely normal. He was now rambling, agitated and unsteady on his feet. An empty bottle of tablets, half a bottle of whisky and a suicide note were found on the kitchen table. On the way to hospital in the ambulance the man had a generalized seizure. There was a past history of psychiatric illness, and previous serious overdoses.

On examination:

- Drowsy. Apyrexial
- Tachycardia 130/min, blood pressure 90/60 mmHg
- Gag reflex intact
- Confused speech
- Eyes open to verbal command, ataxic but purposeful limb movements
- Dilated, reactive pupils
- Fundi normal
- No neck stiffness
- No rash
- Generalized hyperflexia, but no focal neurological signs
- Extensor plantar responses
- Chest clear
- Abdomen soft – palpable bladder to the umbilicus

Questions

1 What were the tablets?
2 What is your immediate management of this patient?

Answers

1 The most likely drugs to give rise to this clinical picture are the tricyclic antidepressants. The toxic side effects of this group of drugs are due to their anticholinergic, cerebral and cardiodepressant actions. Common findings are therefore dilated pupils, dry skin, sinus tachycardia, hallucinations and urinary retention which may all occur as a result of the anticholinergic effect. Altered consciousness, coma, convulsions and brisk reflexes are due to the cerebral effects and the cardiodepressant action may give rise to hypotension. In addition, a wide variety of rhythm disturbances including degrees of atrioventricular block, ventricular ectopics and ventricular tachycardia may occur.

These drugs account for over 300 deaths per year in England and Wales. A combination of metabolic acidosis, respiratory depression, hypotension and malignant rhythm disturbances are the major contributing factors to death in these patients.

2 This patient has altered consciousness. Immediate management should be in accordance with the guidelines listed on p. 212, concerning the management of the comatose patient.

In addition, the following are necessary;

- Additional history from the flatmate.
- Gastric lavage. The anticholinergic effect of the tricyclics delays gastric emptying and lavage can be helpful up to 12 h after ingestion of tricyclic antidepressant drugs.

Table 7   How to perform gastric lavage

1 If unconscious, or absent gag reflex the airway needs protecting with a cuffed endotracheal tube. *Note:* patients with altered consciousness should be assessed by the anaesthetist prior to the procedure
2 Place the patient in the left semi-prone position head down, and attach a pulse oximeter to measure oxygen saturation
3 Pass a wide bore orogastric tube: test aspirate to confirm position, and save a sample for toxicology
4 Pour down warmed water in 500 ml aliquots then siphon this out into a bucket. Continue until aspirate is clear
5 Before removing the tube instill charcoal.

Lavage is indicated when more than 750 mg of tricyclics are taken (adult) (see Table 7).

- Activated charcoal: to gain maximum benefit from activated charcoal, 10 parts charcoal to one part poison is necessary. Therefore it is most effective when it has to absorb substances which are toxic in small amounts such as the tricyclics. A 50 g bolus should be run down the gastric tube when the lavage is complete. Repeat doses of charcoal at 4-hourly intervals may be beneficial at preventing further absorption, presumably by interrupting the enterohepatic circulation.

The acute complications of poisoning should be recognized early and treated promptly. These include:

Hypotension. When the systolic blood pressure drops below 90 mmHg, colloid should be administered. As patients are not hypovolaemic, care should be taken if the hypotension has not responded to a litre of fluid, and further administration should be performed with central venous pressure monitoring. Ionotropes such as dobutamine may be necessary if there is persistent hypotension.

Convulsions. A single convulsion should be terminated with diazepam. Repetitive convulsion however should be treated with phenytoin, at a dose 10–20 mg/kg.

Arrhythmias. Prolongation of the 'QRS' complex and a tachycardia are both suggestive of cardiotoxicity. All symptomatic and all ventricular tachyarrhythmias should be treated with direct current shock. If resistant to electrical cardioversion then the use of phenytoin or amiodarone should be considered (as lignocaine, disopyramide and procainamide are contraindicated). Bradyarrhythmias may necessitate cardiac pacing.

Metabolic acidosis. Metabolic acidosis is common, and exacerbated by the respiratory depression and CO_2 retention. Correction of hypoventilation initially may help, but bicarbonate may be necessary for persisting severe acidosis.

The regional poisons centre should be contacted for advice when serious overdoses give rise to intractable complications. The patient should be referred to the medical team for further management.

Outcome

This man was admitted to a high dependency unit. He developed a bradycardia which was unresponsive to drug therapy and consequently needed a pacing wire. Recovery was complicated by acute tubular necrosis due to a period of unrelieved hypotension.

On recovery he was transferred to the local psychiatric hospital for treatment of his depression.

Further notes

Acute confusional states

The diagnosis of an acute confusional state is made when there is evidence of recent onset of clouding of consciousness and disorientation. The degree of confusion can vary from the incomprehensible patient to subtle changes in the patient's mental state which may not be immediately obvious unless carefully sought.

In practice, acute confusion is most common in the elderly and is often the result of organ failure (respiratory, cardiac, renal), sepsis, an acute neurological insult (cerebrovascular accident), or a metabolic disturbance (hypoglycaemia, hyponatraemia, or adverse drug effects). However, the differentiation between acute and acute-on-chronic organic brain syndromes can be difficult in the elderly, and the history from a carer is most helpful.

In the young, drugs and alcohol are the usual precipitants of acute confusion. There are however a number of serious conditions which should always be included in the differential diagnosis of any patient with an acute confusional state.

These include

1 *Hypoglycaemia.* This condition is readily treatable, and a blood sugar should be urgently performed on all confused patients (see Case 23).

Cautionary tale
An elderly woman presented with acute confusion and a left-sided weakness. She was referred to the medical team as a cerebrovascular accident. The medical houseman gave her glucose i.v. with resolution of the neurological signs and the confusional state.

2 *Drug intoxication/overdose*

- Alcohol: acute intoxication, Korsakoff/Wernicke's encephalopathy
- Psychotropic drugs
- Anticholinergics
- L-dopa
- Solvent abuse
- Amphetamines, LSD, psilocybin mushrooms

3 *Drug withdrawal*

- Alcohol: delirium tremens
- Opiates
- Benzodiazepines

Cautionary tale
A woman presented with an array of bizarre symptoms, and appeared confused. She complained of photophobia, a metallic taste in her mouth, odd sensations as if being covered in cobwebs, hyperacusis and hyperosmia. She was unsteady on her feet and had the illusion of seeing large cracks in the floor.

On examination she was anxious, agitated and paranoid. She had recently run out of diazepam, which she had been taking continuously for the past 4 years and she was felt to be suffering from acute benzodiazepine withdrawal, as many of her symptoms are characteristic of this state.

4 *Cerebral insult*

- Postictal
- Post head injury
- Meningitis
- Subarachnoid haemorrhage (see p. 1)
- Transient global amnesia
- Cerebral infarct
- Encephalitis

Cautionary tales
1 A 56-year-old woman was found muttering outside the office in which she worked unable to negotiate the revolving door to enter the building. She was rambling and was brought to the Accident and Emergency department. She then had a generalized seizure. A CT scan demonstrated a large frontal cerebral infarction.
2 A pregnant woman of 31 was brought by her husband who was worried by his wife's increasing confusion over the last 12 h. It was not obvious at first when assessing her mental state that she was confused, as she answered the questions appropriately. She could not however remember the expected date of delivery of the baby, nor how many children she already had. She was ultimately diagnosed as having herpes simplex encephalitis.

Mental test score

The mental test score, a brief psychometric test is valuable in assessing the acutely confused patient. It provides an objective measure of aspects of cognitive impairment which will confirm the impression of confusion.

Below is the mental test score.

1 Age
2 Time (to nearest hour)
3 Address for recall at end of test, e.g. 42 Gower Street
4 Year
5 Name of hospital
6 Recognition of two people (doctor, nurse)
7 Date of birth
8 Years of the First World War (or other notable event appropriate to the patient)
9 Name of present Monarch
10 Count backwards, from 20 to 1.

The score is expressed out of ten.

Reference

Henry, J. and Volans, G. (eds) (1984) *ABC of poisoning*. BMJ Publications, London

Case 60

A 30-year-old woman presented to Accident and Emergency with the sudden onset of severe left-sided chest pain. She described it as a 'stabbing' type of pain. It started while she was sitting reading the newspaper, was centred around her left nipple, made her sweat and it was worse with inspiration and walking. Specific movements, however, did not affect the pain. The severe component of the pain lasted 90 min, during which time her breathing became laboured and she felt dizzy and lightheaded. The pain then subsided, leaving her with a dull ache. There had been no recent 'cough or cold' symptoms or significant past medical history. She did not smoke, though she did take the oral contraceptive pill. Her father had died of a heart attack aged 65 years. The only other history which was relevant was that she had been decorating the house at the weekend and felt that she might have 'overdone it'.

On examination:

- She was anxious, not distressed
- Pyrexial 37.8°C

- Pulse 88/min, blood pressure 110/70 mmHg, respiratory rate 20/min
- No chest wall tenderness could be elicited
- Chest was clear
- No rubs
- Heart sounds normal
- Abdomen soft
- Calves normal, no obvious deep venous thrombosis but there was a small area of superficial tenderness in the mid calf.

Questions

1 What are the possible diagnoses?
2 What investigations would you perform?
3 What is your management?

Answers

1 Possible diagnoses

The possible diagnoses include the following.

Pneumothorax (or pneumomediastinum): a spontaneous pneumothorax could account for the pain and shortness of breath in this woman. Small and moderate-sized leaks can be difficult to detect clinically and a chest radiograph is necessary to make the diagnosis.

Musculoskeletal pain: to be convinced that chest pain is arising from the thoracic cage, one should be able to reproduce the pain exactly by clinical examination. The chest wall should be palpated, and compressed and the patient asked to do stretching and rotational exercises. However, the ability to reproduce the pain by palpation should be interpreted with caution particularly when the history is suggestive of an alternative diagnosis.

Pericarditis: pericarditis should always be considered in the differential diagnosis of any patient who presents with pleuritic chest pain. A typical history, the nature of the pain, a pericardial rub, and ST changes in the ECG should all be sought.

Pleurisy: pleural involvement from an infective or inflammatory process may give rise to a pleuritic pain of sudden onset. Pleuritic pain is exacerbated by deep inspiration and patients often change their respiratory pattern, taking more frequent and shallower breaths to avoid this. Being aware of the change in respiratory pattern and anxiety gives rise to the associated dyspnoea. There may be a history of a prodromal illness, clinical signs or radiographic changes compatible with consolidation which would be suggestive of an infective cause, however, when the pain arises suddenly in an otherwise well patient, the possibility of pulmonary embolus needs to be entertained.

Pulmonary embolus: the clinical diagnosis of pulmonary embolus can be very difficult. The classical triad of chest pain, dyspnoea and haemoptysis occurs in a minority (less than 20%) of patients. Patients frequently attend the Accident and Emergency department with pleuritic pain, and pulmonary embolus should always be considered in the differential diagnosis. Branch and McNeil (1983) studied 97 patients (all under 40 years) who presented with acute pleuritic chest pain, in whom obvious causes such as pneumonia, pneumothorax, pericarditis and musculoskeletal pain had been excluded. They all were fully investigated including ventilation and perfusion scanning. A specific diagnosis was arrived at in the majority of the 97 cases. They were:

Viral or idiopathic pleurisy	53%
Pulmonary embolus	21%
Pneumonia	18%
Others	8%

Interestingly, in this study the temperature, respiratory rate and the mean arterial Po_2 failed to differentiate between the two groups of patients with either viral/idiopathic pleurisy or pulmonary embolism. However, they did find a positive correlation between the presence of a pulmonary embolus and a history of thrombo-occlusive disease, or risk factors for the same, the presence of phlebitis on examination or a pleural effusion on the chest radiograph.

The Accident and Emergency senior house officer will have to manage many patients with pleuritic-type chest pain. The majority will have either an obvious cause after clinical examination and radiography, or suspected viral/idiopathic pleurisy. However, when the diagnosis is not obvious, pulmonary embolus should always be borne in mind.

All patients with a significant history will need to be investigated. Pulmonary angiography is the gold standard, however, ventilation perfusion scanning is commonly used as a screening investigation.

An electrocardiogram, chest radiograph and arterial blood gases may provide useful information, although normal results do not exclude the diagnosis.

The risk factors, common clinical findings, and abnormalities in investigations associated with a pulmonary embolus are listed below.

History

a Risk factors of thrombo-occlusive venous disease.

   i Following surgery – risk depends upon length and type of procedure.

   ii Trauma – injuries involving pelvis and legs, or major burns including immobilization in plaster of Paris.

iii Prolonged immobilization – usually associated with chronic medical conditions.
iv Pregnancy, puerperium and the oral contraceptive pill.
v Underlying malignancy.
b Past history of pulmonary embolus or deep-vein thrombosis.
c Typical symptoms. Pleuritic chest pain associated with dyspnoea, haemoptysis, cough, sweating and apprehension.

Clinical features

a Raised respiratory rate >16/min.
b Presence of a tachycardia.
c Elevated venous pressure.
d Pleural rub.

Investigations

a Electrocardiogram. ECG changes are common but usually transient. The commonest findings, apart from a tachycardia, are non-specific 'T' wave changes in the anterior chest leads. Atrial fibrillation is found in approximately 18% of patients. Evidence of right axis deviation or right bundle branch block, P pulmonale, or the finding of an S wave in lead I, a Q wave in lead III, and T wave inversion in lead III, are all suggestive but occur in a minority of cases.
b Chest radiograph. The chest radiograph is often normal in the early stages or if abnormal, this is often only appreciated retrospectively.

- Typical wedge shape of a pulmonary infarct
- Increased radiolucency of part of one lung field
- Elevated hemidiaphragm
- Plate atelectasis

c Arterial blood gases.
Low P_aO_2. Any value lower than 12 kPa should be considered abnormal in a patient without pre-existing cardiopulmonary disease. Values below 10 kPa are to be expected with major pulmonary embolus.
Low $P_aCO_2 < 4.5$ kPa.
   Although there are alternative explanations for clinical findings and abnormal investigations, in a patient with pleuritic chest pain with a combination of the above factors, a pulmonary embolus needs to be excluded.

2 Investigations

Investigations in this patient were:

- Electrocardiogram: rate 80/min, T wave inversion in II, III, AVF. No other significant abnormality.

- Chest radiograph: normal. No pneumothorax or consolidation
- Arterial blood gases
    P_aO_2 10.8 kPa
    P_aCO_2 4.1 kPa
    pH 7.38

3 Management

This 30-year-old woman presented with pleuritic type chest pain, for which no obvious cause could be found. She was taking the oral contraceptive pill and had an area of superficial thrombophlebitis on her leg. Both are risk factors for pulmonary embolus. The ECG demonstrated a right axis and non-specific inferior T wave changes, and blood gases revealed unexplained hypoxia. A pulmonary embolus needs to be excluded. This patient should be referred for a V/Q scan.

Outcome

An NSAID helped the pain which settled within 48 h. A ventilation/perfusion scan demonstrated a matched defect in the left lung. A chest radiograph 48 h later demonstrated an area of focal consolidation for which antibiotics were prescribed. There was clinical and radiographic improvement over the next 2 weeks.

The diagnosis was pneumonia.

Cautionary tale
A man of 68 presented with a week's history of dyspnoea. He had initially noticed that he had become increasingly short of breath on exertion, but not at rest. However, for the last two nights he had awoken during the night with shortness of breath, associated with intermittent stabbing chest pain. He was a non-smoker, had no risk factors for ischaemic heart disease, and had been generally fit and well until a week ago. In the past, however, he had had a deep vein thrombosis (DVT) 18 years ago which had been treated with warfarin for 6 months. This had left him with a swollen right leg ever since.

On examination, apart from a tachycardia of 105, there was no abnormality in the cardiovascular system. Auscultation of the chest revealed crepitations at the left base. His right leg was swollen below the knee, but non-tender. He confirmed that the leg had not changed in any way recently and it did not give rise to any symptoms. A chest radiograph was normal, there being no evidence of heart failure and an ECG confirmed the tachycardia but was otherwise normal. Blood gases were not performed.

A diagnosis of incipient heart failure was made and the patient was commenced upon a diuretic and discharged. Two days later, the patient returned in a collapsed state with constant dyspnoea, hypotension and syncope whenever he sat up. He had vomited once that morning which was described as 'coffee grounds'. An initial diagnosis of acute gastrointestinal haemorrhage was made. This was rapidly changed to acute massive pulmonary embolus when the central venous pressure was found to be grossly elevated. The patient died within 2 h of presentation. On reflection, the diagnosis of pulmonary embolus would have been made if it had considered initially.

Reference

Branch, W. T. and McNeil, B. J. (1983) Analysis of the differential diagnosis and assessment of pleuritic chest pain in young adults. *American Journal of Medicine*, **75**, 671

Case 61

A 22-year-old American woman complained of right iliac fossa pain for the past 6 h. The pain was constant in nature and radiated through to her back and to her upper right thigh. It was similar in many respects to her normal period pain, but was more severe. Her period had started that morning. She had vomited with the pain, but there were no other symptoms. In particular, there were no urinary symptoms of frequency or dysuria, and her bowels had been normal. There had been no obvious vaginal discharge.

She had stopped taking the oral contraceptive pill 4 months ago, and her periods had been regular until 6 weeks previously when they had become erratic. Her cycle was normally 5/28, but during the last 6 weeks she had bled on four separate occasions, approximately 2 weeks apart. On two occasions this had been as heavy as normal but the other two were very light and lasted for only 2 days.

She denied feeling pregnant, but admitted to having unprotected intercourse 2 months ago.

There was no other relevant gynaecological history, she had never had pelvic inflammatory disease, an IUCD, or been pregnant. She was otherwise fit and well.

On examination:

- Apyrexial
- Well
- Pulse 96/min, blood pressure 110/70 mmHg
- Chest clear
- Heart sounds normal
- Abdomen: tender in the right lower quadrant. No guarding or rebound. Bowel sounds normal. Rectal examination normal
- Pelvic examination: vulva normal. Cervical examination painful. Very tender in the right fornix. Left fornix non-tender. Swabs taken

The rest of the examination was normal.

Questions

1 What is the differential diagnosis?
2 What is your management?

Answers

1 Your differential diagnosis should include:

Ectopic pregnancy: rupture of an ectopic pregnancy can be fatal. The diagnosis should always be considered in all women in the child-bearing years who present with lower abdominal pain. The unilateral pelvic tenderness and cervical excitation found in this woman support the diagnosis and urinary or serum beta-HCG estimation is necessary.

(It is imperative that a sensitive pregnancy test is performed on all such patients to exclude this diagnosis.)

Ovarian cyst accident: ovarian cysts may rupture, bleed, or undergo torsion. Torsion is uncommon, and usually occurs in ovaries which are abnormal. The usual pathology being a dermoid or a simple cyst, but a significant proportion will be found to be malignant.

Patients normally present with acute lower abdominal pain, associated with nausea and vomiting. There may be a history of previous pain, which lasted for hours or sometimes days, and a history of menstrual irregularity. The pain is typically a severe dull ache with sharp exacerbations.

Examination reveals a palpable tender adnexal mass in over 80% of patients, and cervical excitation.

If torsion goes unrecognized, necrosis of the organ can lead to peritonitis and shock. Ultrasound can be helpful in making the diagnosis, though laparoscopy is necessary for confirmation.

In this woman the history of constant pain, with the pelvic findings suggests that torsion of the right ovary is a possibility.

Dysmenorrhoea: dysmenorrhoea is common, and being a recurrent phenomenon, women are very aware of the nature of their symptoms and therefore do not usually present to the Accident and Emergency department with simple dysmenorrhoea. This should be diagnosis of exclusion rather than the principle diagnosis when assessing any woman with lower abdominal pain.

The pain tends to be most severe on the day when the blood loss is the greatest, and although this typically is the first day, it is not necessarily so. Conditions such as chronic pelvic infection should be excluded as it can exacerbate the pelvic pain associated with menstruation. Pelvic inflammatory disease gives rise to bilateral symptoms and signs though pain on one particular side may predominate.

Appendicitis: the diagnosis should always be considered, if only to be excluded. In this woman the pain started with a period, is constant in site, and radiates outside of the abdomen (thigh) all which make the diagnosis unlikely. *Cervical excitation* and *adnexal tenderness* would be *unlikely* to be due to an acutely inflamed appendix. (See diagnosis of appendicitis, p. 9.)

However, differentiating appendicitis from pelvic pathology can be very difficult. Laparoscopy can be very helpful when there is diagnostic difficulty.

Ureteric colic: again this is a diagnosis which should be considered briefly when patients present with atypical right lower quadrant pain. Urinanalysis and a plain abdominal radiograph are useful screening tests (the latter if she is not pregnant).

2 The management in this case includes:

a Excluding ectopic pregnancy by performing a sensitive pregnancy test. (Although very occasionaly even a sensitive beta-HCG may be negative in the presence of an ectopic pregnancy.)
b Refer the patient to the gynaecological team for an opinion and further investigations (ultrasound).

Outcome

The beta-HCG was negative. The gynaecology registrar confirmed the pelvic findings. She believed that an 'ovarian accident' was likely. However, an ultrasound examination failed to demonstrate the right ovary. Laparoscopy was normal. The pain settled spontaneously and the patient was discharged home. The diagnosis being dysmenorrhoea.

Reference

London, J. D. O. Chapter 42 in *Hamilton Bailey's Emergency Surgery*, 11th edn. Wright, Bristol, 448

Appendix

Emergency management

Consciousness is maintained by an interaction between the reticular activating system in the brainstem and the cerebral hemispheres. Altered consciousness or coma is produced when there is an interruption in this 'circuit'.

The aims of immediate management in the comatose patient are to treat life-threatening emergencies and limit further deterioration.

Patients who are semiconscious or comatose as a result of trauma need immediate management by the trauma team (surgeons and the anaesthetist). In patients in whom there is no history of, or evidence of trauma, always entertain this possibility early in the differential diagnosis.

Senior help and an anaesthetist should be called immediately for all comatose patients, and the patient managed in the resuscitation area.

Immediate management consists of:

Airway: in any patient with altered consciousness the potential for airway obstruction is high. Clear and control the airway:
suction
'chinlift' manoeuvre
oropharyngeal or nasopharyngeal airway if tolerated
60% oxygen by Venturi mask
gag reflex is absent then the airway needs protecting – pass an endotracheal tube.

Breathing: if the respiratory rate is less than 10/min assisted ventilation may be necessary. If the patient becomes apnoeic pass an endotracheal tube. Ventilate with 100% oxygen. Remember give naloxone if:
i   Intubation is necessary or respiratory rate <10/min
ii Pin-point pupils are present
iii 'Needle track' marks are evident

Circulation: connect the patient to a cardiac monitor. Measure the blood pressure. Establish venous access. Exclude hypoglycaemia – give 50 ml 50% dextrose if the BM stix <4 mmol/l.
Take blood for:
full blood count
urea and electrolytes
blood sugar
toxicology
arterial blood gas analysis
Connect the patient to the pulse oximeter

If the patient is hypotensive but the pressure is >90 mmHg tip the end of the bed; <90 mmHg infuse colloid and measure the central venous pressure.

Catheterization is necessary for all unconscious patients.

Disability: assess the level of consciousness with the aid of the Glasgow coma score. Remember patients scoring 14–9 are said to have altered consciousness and those scoring 8 or less as being in coma.

Exposure: completely undress the patient. The clothes should be searched for useful information such as medical cards, drugs, next of kin etc.

Having stabilized the patient and maintained vital functions the history should be sought from attending relatives, friends, ambulance staff and the general practitioner if necessary.

A thorough head-to-toe examination of the patient should then take place to look for evidence of precipitating factors such as head injury, infection, drug abuse or vascular catastrophes.

Particular attention should be paid to:

- Level of consciousness (Glasgow coma score)
- Assessment of brainstem function
- Focal neurological signs

Bedside assessment of brainstem function

a *Pupillary response*: the size, shape, and response to light of the pupils should be noted. An understanding of the common changes in the pupillary reflexes is important in localization of lesions. For example, with lesions that directly affect the brainstem (pontine haemorrhage) the pupillary responses are abnormal from the outset, whereas in metabolic coma (e.g. drug overdose, alcohol) and coma produced by widespread cerebral hemisphere dysfunction (e.g. postictal) they are preserved. Common variants of pupillary changes are shown in the illustration below.

b *Eye movements*: many patients in coma have roving, or dyscongulate eye movements when observed; these are common and are of no particular significance.

The oculocephalic response (doll's-head eye movements) provides useful information about the oculomotor and vestibular components of brainstem function. The response is elicited by quickly turning the head to one side, while holding the eye lids open, and observing eye movements. Initially the eyes will not move with the head and appear to be 'left behind'. Slowly they will return to the central position in relationship to the head. The response will be absent in patients with depressed brainstem function and patients not in coma (i.e. physiologically awake).

		Size and response	Cause
		Normal	e.g. metabolic coma psychogenic unresponsiveness
		Widely dilated	e.g. post cardiac arrest
		Minimal or no reaction to light	drugs – atropine adrenaline
		Pin-point unreactive	e.g. opiate overdose pontine haemorrhage
		Unilateral dilated pupil, sluggish response	uncal herniation
		Progressing to complete III nerve palsy	
		Mid-position unreactive	e.g. midbrain damage

(Adapted from Spingings, D. and Chambers, J. (1990) *Acute Medicine*. Blackwell Scientific Publications, Oxford)

The oculovestibular (caloric) test. This is a much more potent stimulus to the brainstem function than the oculocephalic reflex, but is more time consuming to perform and often unsuitable for Accident and Emergency assessments. It is useful however in one instance, that of psychogenic unresponsiveness. Having first ensured that the ear drums are intact, the head is inclined at 30° to the trunk, and the external auditory canal of one ear is irrigated with ice cold water while the eyes are held open. In those comatose patients with an intact vestibular component there is a tonic deviation of the eyes to the irrigated ear, while in patients not in coma it produces nystagmus and vomiting. (The quick phase is away from the irrigated side.) There is no movement of the eyes when brainstem function is lost.

c *Corneal reflexes* are usually preserved in coma. In the absence of drugs, the loss of this reflex is a very poor sign.

d *Respiratory patterns*: alterations in brainstem function produce a variety of respiratory patterns, which may help to localize the lesion. In practice, however, they are of limited value.

   i Eupnoeic – normal, e.g. postictal metabolic coma.

   ii Periodic breathing (Cheynes-Stokes), e.g. lesions to the diencephalon, though there are many non-cerebral causes of periodic breathing including heart failure.

iii Central neurogenic hyperventilation, e.g. lesion to the midbrain or upper pons.

iv Ataxia breathing (slow and irregular), lesions to the medulla.

v Deep sighing respiration (Kussmaul), associated with a metabolic acidosis.

Motor function

When assessing motor response to pain, tone, and deep tendon reflexes you are looking for asymmetry. Asymmetrical signs with intact brainstem reflexes suggest a focal hemispheric lesion. Whereas focal signs with absent brainstem reflexes are suggestive of a lesion in the posterior fossa. Information gained by assessing the brainstem reflexes can be very valuable in localizing the lesion, and to help select which patients will need immediate further investigation, e.g. CT scanning.

Coma can be caused by the broad pathophysiological insults listed below. Some common causes are listed, and an indication of the typical signs are included.

References

Plum, F. and Posner, J. B. (1980) *The Diagnosis of Stupor and Coma.* F. A. Davis Co., Philadelphia

Springings, D. and Chambers, J. (1990) *Acute Medicine.* Blackwell Scientific Publications, Oxford

Cause of coma – for emergency management

Pathophysiology	Common causes	Typical signs	Additional notes
Global disturbance due to metabolic imbalance	Drug overdose Hypoglycaemia Hepatic } Renal } Failure Respiratory } Hyponatremia	Normal pupillary responses Normal or absent eye movement depending on depth of coma Cheyne-Stokes respiration Symmetrical, hypotonic limb signs	Always exclude hypoglycaemia Consider naloxone in all comatose patients
Widespread hemispheric disturbance	Head injury Postictal Meningitis Encephalitis Hypertensive crisis Subarachnoid haemorrhage	Normal pupil responses Eye movements normal Respiration normal Symmetrical limb signs	Signs of meningeal irritation may be absent in the comatose patient. Signs of sepsis usually present. Convulsions or myoclonus may occur
Distortion of brainstem by an expanding supratentorial mass	Cerebral infarct/haemorrhage Extradural/subdural haemorrhage Abscess Tumour	Progressive development of unilateral third nerve signs. Progressive development of abnormal respiratory pattern and other brainstem signs as compression of brainstem continues. Asymmetrical limb signs Sequential loss of signs	Patients with subdural and particularly extradural haematomas may not have had a significant head injury

Distortion of brainstem by subtentorial masses or vascular catastrophe	*Intrinsic* Brainstem haemorrhage/infarct *Extrinsic* Cerebellar haematoma Abscess Subdura haemorrhage	Brainstem signs present from outset Pin-point pupils, eye movement abnormal Cranial nerve palsies Asymmetrical limb signs	May be a history of previous brainstem dysfunction with diplopia, vertigo, vomiting, ataxia Coma is of sudden onset
Psychogenic unresponsiveness	Conversion hysteria Malingering Neuroses	Inconsistent signs Lids closed actively Pupils equal and reactive Oculocephalics inconsistent Oculovestibular ataxia and vomiting Respiration normal or hyperventilation May simulate focal limb signs	This is a diagnosis of exclusion All patients should be seen by the psychiatrist

Index